SOLUTION-FOCUSED INTERVIEWING

Applying Positive Psychology
A Manual for Practitioners

Too often doctors, therapists, and social workers ask "what's the problem?" rather than "what are you looking for?" Ronald E. Warner's *Solution-Focused Interviewing* is a practical guide for practitioners that uses a solution-driven and strength-based approach to empower clients and help them to find lasting solutions to their problems and effect real change in their lives.

In solution-focused interviewing, practitioners build empathy by first asking clients questions about their goals, resources, and strengths. This important step is the basis of a three-part therapeutic process that assists clients in setting realistic goals and building a plan to achieve them.

Based on Warner's extensive clinical experience and therapy workshops conducted over more than two decades, *Solution-Focused Interviewing* is the first skill-development manual based on this innovative tri-phase approach to counselling and applied positive psychology.

RONALD E. WARNER is a practising psychologist, a professor emeritus at Ryerson University, and the director of the Solution-Focused Counselling Program at the University of Toronto.

RONALD E. WARNER

Solution-Focused Interviewing

Applying Positive Psychology
A Manual for Practitioners

UNIVERSITY OF TORONTO PRESS
Toronto Buffalo London

© University of Toronto Press 2013
Toronto Buffalo London
www.utppublishing.com
Printed in the U.S.A.

Reprinted 2015

ISBN 978-1-4426-4738-1 (cloth)
ISBN 978-1-4426-1549-6 (paper)

Printed on acid-free, 100% post-consumer recycled paper.

Library and Archives Canada Cataloguing in Publication

Warner, Ronald Earl, 1938–, author
Solution-focused interviewing : applying positive psychology,
a manual for practitioners / Ronald E. Warner.

Includes bibliographical references.
ISBN 978-1-4426-4738-1 (bound).   ISBN 978-1-4426-1549-6 (pbk.)

1. Positive psychology – Handbooks, manuals, etc.   I. Title.

BF204.6.W27 2013   150.19′88   C2013-903891-4

University of Toronto Press acknowledges the financial assistance to its
publishing program of the Canada Council for the Arts and the Ontario
Arts Council.

  Canada Council   Conseil des Arts
for the Arts   du Canada

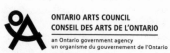

University of Toronto Press acknowledges the financial support of the
Government of Canada through the Canada Book Fund for its publishing
activities.

Contents

Acknowledgments

This manual is dedicated to the memory of Insoo Kim Berg and Steve de Shazer, from whom I learned so much about the conducting of brief helping interviews and the practice of staying positive by focusing on people's strengths and best intentions. The passing of these two extraordinary pioneers marks the end of an era for all of us who knew them and benefited from their tireless efforts to make a more humane world.

I would like to acknowledge a former student, Jason Kelly, who boldly strived to make a difference, but whose full potential was cut short by his premature death.

Finally, I would like to thank my partner, Janet, not only for her encouragement, advice, and editing of the first draft of the manuscript, but also (and more importantly) for supporting and inspiring me in my professional and personal life.

PART ONE

Background

Chapter One

Introduction and Overview

Purpose of the Manual

Welcome to the study of solution-focused interviewing, an effective, safe, and brief approach to helping others. This approach utilizes client strengths and resources rather than expert-directed problem discussions and answers. There are basically two approaches to conducting helping interviews. What distinguishes the dialogue of these two different approaches is the nature of the questions asked. Questions that are directed at fostering understanding of what is wrong, and particularly any kind of problem exploration or analysis, can be described as problem-focused and deficit-based. Strength-based questions, in contrast, are directed at discovering what the client[1] wants to do about the problem, and at expanding the client's awareness of the options available. Further, strength-based questions are directed at uncovering client strengths and resources that can be utilized to build solutions to the problem. How to formulate and deliver strength-based questions – to facilitate the transition from "problem talk" to "solution talk" – is the focus of this manual.

Solution-focused interviewing is an adaptation of solution-focused brief therapy. It was originally intended for non-clinical-psychology (or non-psychotherapy) applications, but its value in both clinical and non-clinical settings is now thoroughly established. The information contained within this manual is directed to healthcare practitioners and the

---

1 *Client* is meant to be a generic "helpee" term that applies to patient, student, employee, friend, or family member.

wide variety of other helping professionals whose scope of practice or job description includes some form of general counselling or advising. The manual is also intended for use by participants in the solution-focused interviewing workshops that I conduct.

In an effort to help my workshop participants acquire skills more quickly, I have for the last few years requested that they complete some pre-workshop reading. This pre-workshop preparation has, on the whole, resulted in more advanced workshops. When less time is spent discussing theoretical issues, more time is left to discuss and practice client applications. Specifically, I have noticed that prepared partici-pants demonstrate better interviewing skill in both the role-playing exercises and the small-group practice sessions. This manual is an ex-panded form of the pre-workshop reading I formerly assigned. It in-corporates the workshop preparation and reading suggestions and it provides more detailed information about how to use solution-focused interviewing techniques effectively.

Workshop Preparation: To Participants

Set out below are suggestions to workshop participants on how to pre-pare for training.

- Review the "Questions for Reflection" section below and keep these questions in mind while reading the next chapter. The answers to these questions and the important practice issues they raise will be discussed at the workshop. Beginning to think about these ques-tions before the workshop will provide a basic understanding and a stronger foundation for the development of your solution-building skills.
- Read chapter 2, "Fast Track to Beginning Practice," carefully. This brief chapter provides information about the essentials of the ap-proach. It will help you understand what solution-focused inter-viewing is all about. To obtain the most from your training, and to be able to apply the solution-focused techniques effectively by the end of the workshop, consider how you would answer the follow-ing questions.

Questions for Reflection

1 What is the difference between solution-building and problem-focused intervention questions?

2 What are negative goals and how do we reframe them as positive goals?
3 What are the three characteristics of well-formed goals?
4 What is the purpose of each component of the tri-phase model of solution building?
5 Considering your interviewing style, how would you rank the five primary intervention questions in terms of anticipated ease of use with your clients?

- Finally, give some thought to selecting a goal for your own personal development. Workshop participants will have opportunities to work on personal goals in small-group practice sessions. There will be opportunities for interested participants to take part in my solution-building demonstration interviews.

Overview of the Manual

Part One: Background

Chapter 2 provides a brief overview of solution-focused interviewing. It is intended as a "fast-track" introduction. Chapter 3, "Human Development and Models of Psychology," reflects my research interests and frames the solution-focused approach in the context of strength-based psychology, including the emerging field of "positive psychology." The contents of this chapter will be most relevant to those with an academic interest in psychology. I do not usually enter into detailed discussions about these topics in my workshops because of time constraints. Appendix D provides a description of how I came to adopt the solution-focused therapy model in my professional practice.

Part Two: The Tri-Phase Model for Learning Solution-Focused Skills

Chapter 4 offers an overview of the solution-focused brief therapy model. Chapters 5 to 7 represent the "how to" portion of the manual. In these chapters, you will find a detailed description of how to ask strength-based questions – questions that will promote "solution talk" and empower clients to take action, to do something to improve their situation, and to build solutions to what is troubling them.

Readers are encouraged to take a "bits-and-pieces" approach to using this manual. Solution-building questions, being strength-based, have considerably less risk – compared to problem-focused questions

– of opening up emotionally laden areas. And strength-based questions are most often intrinsically helpful – meaning that the question itself is helpful to the client and its helpfulness does not depend on the questioner's understanding of the strategies, theory, or model. Therefore, the reader need not start at the beginning of the manual and successively work through each chapter, but rather may pick out those parts that seem most relevant and move on to any other area of interest.

Background of the Author

Dr Ronald E. Warner, psychologist, worked in clinical practice for thirty years as a counsellor at Ryerson University, where he was named professor emeritus in 2001. He is the founding director of the Certificate Program in Solution-Focused Counselling at the Faculty of Social Work, University of Toronto, and for twenty years was an adjunct faculty instructor in the Counselling Psychology Program at the OISE/University of Toronto. He is also the examiner for the solution-focused professional designations offered by the Canadian Council of Professional Certification. From 1998 to 2004 he served as an honorary research fellow in the Centre for Studies in Counselling at the University of Durham, United Kingdom. He has authored more than thirty publications related to the practice of brief therapy.

From his private practice in Kingston, where he resides, he offers solution-focused training throughout southern Ontario and abroad. For the past four years his therapy practice has been focused on treating soldiers suffering from trauma and post-traumatic stress disorder at the Canadian Forces Base Kingston where he established the first Post-Traumatic Growth therapy group.

Chapter Two

Fast Track to Beginning Practice

The Power of Questions

Judge a man by his questions, rather than his answers.

Voltaire

Too often we offer explanations or observations when we should be engaging in inquiry. It may be gratifying to display knowledge and expertise, but our explanations and observations rarely empower the people to whom we are speaking. Questions, on the other hand, have the power and the potential to evoke and transform thought into an energized belief system that can become life-altering. Questions can create new possibilities, new hope and new inspiration that can lead to transformation and higher levels of functioning and fulfilment.

Strength-based questions, when used in solution-focused interviewing, are potent inquiries because they are grounded in our clients' successes, capabilities, and aspirations. Such inquiries lead to an increased experience of optimism and positive feelings. And most important, recent research findings (see chapter 3) demonstrate that positive emotions also increase psychological well-being, future health, and longevity.

Solution-Focused Interviewing: Description

The solution-focused interviewer learns the skills to conduct interviews and discussions in which clients' existing strengths and resources are utilized to help them define their goals and develop solutions to their problems.[1] This interviewing approach addresses solutions rather than problems by emphasizing client strengths, competencies, and possibilities rather than weaknesses, deficits, and limitations. The solution-focused approach differs from the conventional problem-based paradigm in that it de-emphasizes the connection between the problem and its solution. It also emphasizes the importance of client perceptions and de-emphasizes the role of the practitioner as the expert who makes assessments and prescribes interventions (De Jong & Berg, 2008).

Problem Talk Compared to Solution Talk: An Important Distinction

All client interactions, understandably, begin with a discussion of the problem or difficult situation. However, questions directed at acquiring details to gain an understanding of the problem promote problem discussion or, more simply, "problem talk." One of the core skills of the solution-focused approach is to ask questions early in the conversation that facilitate the client making the transition from problem talk – talk about "what's wrong" to solution talk – talk about "what's wanted." All questions can be seen as promoting either problem talk or solution talk. It is important to understand clearly the differences between these two approaches.

Problem Talk: "What's Wrong" – The Traditional Helping Approach

Problem talk is facilitated by questions that encourage expansion on "what's wrong," including questions about the nature, frequency, intensity, duration, and cause of the problem. Exploration of the problem is crucial, according to this paradigm, so that the client and professional can come to an understanding of the difficulty. The underlying assumption here is that resolution to problems develops solely out of insight or knowledge gained from problem discussion. Some helping models (e.g., psychoanalysis) go further and maintain that it is of crucial importance to uncover and explore the "root" cause of the problem. The importance of finding the cause of the problem, for these models, is based on three presuppositions: that all psychosocial problems have a specific cause, that the cause can be identified, and that there is a con-

---

1 This description applies equally to solution-focused brief therapy.

nection between finding the cause and resolving the problem (Walter & Peller, 1992).

Solution Talk: "What's Wanted" – A Paradigm Shift

In contrast to exploring "what's wrong," the solution-focused approach explores what the client wants to do about the specific problem. The interviewer listens sympathetically to the client's statement of the problem, but looks for opportunities to ask questions about what's wanted in order to begin solution talk. Solution talk is promoted by interviewer questions that focus on client successes, strengths, resources, and goals. The interviewer and client explore together a more hopeful vision of a future in which the problem is resolved. In situations where the client is dealing with irreparable loss, the questions explore a future in which the client is coping as well as possible. Before solution talk can progress, the interviewer must first establish good rapport and be perceived as understanding the client and the problem.

The solution-building interview can also be differentiated from the conventional problem-focused interview by the positive ambience of the discussion. Underlying all inquiries directed to the client is the presupposition that clients possess what they need to resolve their difficulties. Strength-based questions – all inquiries that are directed at and emphasize positive attributes – help clients become aware of their capabilities and create this positive atmosphere.

Operational Components of Solution-Focused Interviewing (SFI)

- We do not consider the client's or interviewer's understanding of the problem a necessary condition for the resolution of the difficulty.
- We identify the client's unique personal strengths and resources.
- We explore what the client wants to be different in his or her life – the goal.
- We mobilize strengths and clarify goals to provide the foundation for the interviewer and client to co-construct a solution to the problem that initiated the interview.

Example: Michael's Promotion Interview

MICHAEL: Yesterday I was told that I had made it to the second round of interviews next Tuesday, but – here is what throws me – Mr Jacobs, the senior manager, will be chairing the meeting! He has a reputation of being very critical and tough on employees, and frankly, many of us are intimidated by him. Last night, I hardly slept at all worrying about this – I even had a nightmare about losing it during the interview!

The following are examples of problem-focused questions that are likely to promote extended problem-exploration and problem talk.

Problem-Focused Questions: Examples

- What is it about Mr Jacobs that intimidates you?
- Have you personally had a run-in with him before?
- Does Mr Jacobs remind you of other people in your life who have been critical of you?
- What, specifically, were you thinking about last night that kept you awake and caused a nightmare?

Now, let's look at strength-based questions that promote solution talk and would help Michael to see the strengths and competencies he possesses that will enable him to do well in the upcoming interview.

Solution-Building Questions: Examples

- So you had a first interview that was successful! Can you tell me more about it?
- What do you think you said, or how did you handle yourself so that you convinced the committee to give you another interview?
- Based on that interview and similar situations in which you have been successful, what do you need to do to come across at your best in the upcoming interview?
- If Mr Jacobs asks you a tough question – one that you are not sure how to answer, but you are at your best – how would you like to respond to him?

Any of the above questions will likely begin the process of solution building and goal clarification. These questions will not be very helpful to the client, however, until the "empathy phase" of the interview has been effectively undertaken. The phases of the solution-building interview are explained later in this chapter. But first let's examine the assumptions and principles of SFI.

Guiding Assumptions and Principles of Solution-Focused Interviewing

Accentuate the Positive

This principle is the foundation of the model. It is at the core of all strategies and questions. Focusing on the positive, what is wanted (rather than what is wrong), and emphasizing strengths and resources results in client change and empowerment. An important assumption here is that clients, regardless of their problems or situations, already possess sufficient strengths and resources to build solutions to their psychosocial problems. Problem analysis, exploring what is wrong, is considered counterproductive in this strength-based approach. Our capacity to change is connected to our ability to see things differently (De Jong & Berg, 2008).

Construct Positive Goals

Goals, what the client wants, provide direction for the solution-focused approach. When goals are articulated by clients – goals that are based on what is most important to them – there is enhanced hopefulness and motivation to change. Goals need to be expressed in small, behavioural, and positive terms. Negative goals – stopping or not doing something – are unproductive and need to be reframed. We do this by asking clients what they will be doing when the unwanted behaviour is no longer an issue. As long as clients can be helped to identify what they want, regardless of the nature of the problem or diagnosis, the solution-focused approach can be helpful (Sklare, 2005).

Assume a Not-Knowing, Non-Expert Posture

Clients are considered to be experts on their lives – on what will "work" for them and on what they want for their future. Adopting a not-knowing posture, a posture of genuine curiosity towards clients' successes, strengths, and aspirations instils motivation to change, hope, and empowerment. All questions ought to be framed from this not-knowing, non-expert perspective, a perspective that could be described as one of complimentary curiosity.

Use a Solution-Building Process

The solution-focused practitioner need not be an expert on client problems and their resolution, but must have acquired expertise in the solution-building process. The interviewer's role in solution building can be described as that of a coach asking questions that identify strengths, clarify goals, and highlight values – things that are most important to the client. The strength-based conversation instils hope in clients that they can take responsibility for making the desired positive changes in their lives. This approach is consistent with the notion that all psychological treatment facilitates naturally occurring self-healing processes (Bohart & Tallman, 1999).

The following describes the phases of a solution-building process.

Tri-Phase Model of the Solution-Building Process

During my first decade of teaching the solution-focused model, I emphasized the "drivers" – the five primary intervention questions presented later in this chapter. I noted, however, that students and workshop participants experienced two major difficulties when using these powerful questions. First, there were often difficulties related to the fact that the interviewer did not display adequate understanding of the client's situation – in other words, the interviewer was not sufficiently empathic. The second difficulty related to there being insufficient clarity about what the client wanted – client-generated goals. As a result of these two difficulties, I began teaching the model using a tri-phase approach that conceptualized the interview as being composed of three discrete, but interactive, tasks or phases. I now emphasize the importance of demonstrating empathy to the client before moving into the Goal-Setting (e.g., "What do you want?") and Goal-Striving Phase ("What are your ideas of how to get there?") phases and asking any of the five primary intervention questions. This conceptualization provides a template for engaging the client in a more systematic manner and its adoption has resulted in more rapid acquisition of solution-building skills by novices.

Empathy Phase (1): Establishing Rapport

The challenge of this phase is to demonstrate an understanding of and respect for the client's world view in as brief a time as possible. This is accomplished by employing active listening and reflecting skills. It requires acknowledgment of the client's circumstances and adequate validation of the client's story. The interviewer identifies what and who is important to the client and pays close attention to and compliments the client on perceived strengths, successes, and resources. Note: *Emotions and negative feelings are acknowledged and validated, but not explored or expanded upon by the interviewer.*

In the case of Michael, who is worried about his job promotion interview, an empathy-phase response could be as simple as "This promotion is important to you. I can see why you are concerned." To use another example – that of an open-heart surgery patient who expresses apprehension about her upcoming surgery – an empathic response might be "It is perfectly understandable to be apprehensive about major surgery." Chapter 5 provides an in-depth discussion of the empathy phase of the interview. Once the interviewer has given empathic responses and identified and commented on client strengths or resources, it is time to make the transition to the next phase.

Goal-Setting Phase (2): Providing Direction – "What's Wanted"

In this phase, the interviewer and client define a goal – what the client wants to have happen. Goals are defined in small, behavioural, and positive terms. As the discussion progresses, goals change frequently and the interviewer needs to regularly check with the client to clarify these changes. Asking clients what is it that "tells" them that they can achieve their goals often uncovers strengths, resources, and values that result in enhanced determination and confidence. When goals are explored from a solution-building perspective by using the following three steps, clients often find their motivation increases and the experience is frequently transformative and empowering.

FORMING SOLUTION-FOCUSED GOALS

1. Ask "What's Wanted":

Examples: "How can I help you?" "What would you like to do (or change) about this?" "What is it that you want to have happen here?" "How are you hoping I can help you with this?" With involuntary clients, relationship questions can be very helpful. For example, "What would (the judge, teacher, parent, etc.) say is the reason she sent you to see me?" "What would she think it would be helpful for us to talk about right now?"

2. Inquire about the Impact of Obtaining the Goal:

Examples: "What difference will reaching that goal make in your life?" "How will your relationship with your son be better when he improves his grades?"

3. Assess the Level of Motivation:

Examples: "How important is that goal to you? On a scale of 1 to 10, where 1 represents minimal importance (for now you can live with the status quo) and 10 represents great importance (you need to make significant progress towards achieving the goal now), what number would you assign that goal?" "How did you get to that number?" "Can you think of anything that would increase your motivation to achieve that goal by one half-point on the scale?"

Goal-Striving Phase[2] (3): Determining How to Attain the Goal

The attainment of this phase is facilitated by the groundwork undertaken in the two previous phases. It requires that the client begin to think about the possibility that there are new and better ways to deal with the situation, and to take responsibility for making changes that will turn his or her vision of what's wanted into reality. The goal-striving (and often goal-setting) phase involves the interviewer's skilful use of the following primary intervention questions. Using one or more of these questions challenges clients to begin thinking about how they are going to build a solution to their problem.

The Primary Intervention Questions

1. Exceptions – exceptions to the problem:

Finding exceptions shrinks problems, demonstrates abilities and strengths, and focuses on what is possible. The interviewer inquires

---

2 This third phase was initially called Strategy.

about the times when the client's problem or complaint is absent or minimal and what is different about those times.

2. Outcomes – preferred future:

Here we ask clients about their future when the problem is resolved, or when they are coping with the situation as well as possible. The interviewer gathers as many details as possible about how clients' lives or situations will be different when they are successful. The "miracle question," the most powerful of all the outcome techniques, asks clients to imagine that the problem they are having is miraculously resolved while they are sleeping, and then asks them how they would know in the morning that a miracle had happened.

3. Scaling – goal assessment:

We ask clients about their progress towards achieving the goal or their motivation to achieve the goal. We can employ a scale where 1 represents the worst things have been, and 10 represents when the goal is achieved, or where 1 represents very low motivation to reach the goal and 10 represents maximum motivation to reach it. After clients mention a number, we ask two further questions: "How did you get to that number?" and "What would have to happen for you to move up one half-point on that scale?"

4. Relationship – other opinions:

Here we ask clients how someone else who knows them would answer a particular question. For example, "What would your partner say is different about you when you are handling stress better at the office?"

5. Coping – survival skills:

Here we ask clients about how they deal with setbacks. For example, "How have you managed to cope with this (problem or complaint) as well as you have?" or "What has helped you even a little to get through the day?"

Overview

Empathy Phase (1)
Helping the client to feel understood

Goal-Setting Phase (2)
Providing direction

Goal-Striving Phase (3)
Beginning with client's ideas

Using our client Michael, let's see how a solution-focused interview progresses through the three phases.

MICHAEL: Yesterday I was told that I had made it to the second round of interviews next Tuesday, but – here is what throws me – Mr Jacobs, the senior manager, will be chairing the meeting! He has a reputation of being very critical and tough on employees, and frankly, many of us are intimidated by him. Last night, I hardly slept at all worrying about this – I even had a nightmare about losing it during the interview!

INTERVIEWER: Sounds like this job promotion is pretty important to you and you're nervous about it going well. (*Empathy phase response*)

MICHAEL: Yes it is important. I've been doing this job for five years now and really feel I'm ready to move up. But I'm really afraid of blowing this interview – I've done that before!

INTERVIEWER: I hear you (*Empathy response*), but I'm curious – you had a first interview that was successful. Is that right? Can you tell me about that? (*Empathy phase and highlighting a success*)

MICHAEL: Yes, that interview went very well. I just felt prepared and in control – it was the best interview I ever had!

INTERVIEWER: So is that what you want – your goal is to be really prepared and in control in the next interview? (*Important transition to the goal-setting phase*)

MICHAEL: Oh yes – I really want this job. I feel ready for the additional responsibilities, and frankly, my family could use the additional income. (*The client confirms the goal.*)

INTERVIEWER: Sounds like you're both ready and motivated to have this job. (Reiterates the goal and Michael strongly nods agreement.) So what do you have to do to prepare yourself for this interview? (*Goal-striving phase question*)

MICHAEL: Well, last time I was able to keep myself really positive – well, most of the time – and I wonder if that is why I was able to feel on top in the interview.

INTERVIEWER: Sounds right to me (*Empathy response*). So how were you able to do that – stay positive? (*Goal-striving phase question*)

Other questions might be "What would help you stay positive?" "What is it like for you when you are in a positive mood?" "How did you learn to stay positive?" or "How would you like to handle the tough questions that Mr Jacobs might ask?"

This completes our brief introduction to SFI. The remainder of the manual may be read sequentially, or readers may pick and choose from the following chapters according to what is most relevant to their needs. Part Two of the manual provides detailed information about how to use the tri-phase model in solution-focused interviewing.

Chapter Three

Human Development and Models of Psychology

The greater danger for most of us lies not in setting our aim too high and falling short, but in setting our aim too low and achieving our mark.

Michelangelo

Our unique individual perceptions about human nature profoundly influence our behaviour, sense of well-being, and overall quality of life. No one is spared life-altering, destabilizing experiences. Basic security issues – how safe we feel in the world, how much control we believe we have over our lives, and how best to recover from the "slings and arrows" of the human journey – these are the core issues addressed by the models of psychology. My interest in these issues was a motivating factor in my becoming a psychologist.

Theoretical Orientations

One of the biggest surprises for first-year psychology students, myself included, relates to the fact that not only are there conflicting views on the causes of psychopathology, but that there are also so many competing and conflicting schools or models of psychotherapy treatment – as many as 400! As an undergraduate student in the 1960s studying Freud, psychoanalysis, and the DSM (*Diagnostic and Statistical Manual*), I remember how eager I was to question the first psychiatrist I met about the use of the DSM, and how disappointed and astonished I was when he said it was not useful in his practice. Thus began my long-term interest in theoretical orientations that over the years led me to teaching models of psychology to graduate students, to conducting survey research on the practices of Canadian psychologists and counsellors, and to searching for the model best suited to my practice.

In graduate school, my earlier interest in psychoanalysis was replaced by an interest in Carl Rogers's client-centred therapy (Rogers, 1959) – an approach that represented a radical departure from the medical model. Rogers rejected the "therapist as expert" concept that is central to psychoanalysis, other medically oriented approaches, and most contemporary models. In the client-centred approach, the therapist primarily utilizes the client–therapist relationship as the healing force and refrains from providing any diagnosis, assessment, direction, advice, or opinion, and even refrains from asking any questions. The most recent support for the effectiveness of this approach is a five-year follow-up study by Gibbard & Hanley (2008):

> Person-centred counselling is effective for clients with common mental health problems, such as anxiety and depression. Effectiveness is not limited to individuals with mild to moderate symptoms of recent onset, but extends to people with moderate to severe symptoms of longer duration. (p. 215)

Further support for the healing power of empathic understanding is reflected in the fact that members of the American Psychological Association voted Rogers the most influential psychotherapist of the twentieth century. Second place went to Albert Ellis (cognitive-behavioural psychotherapy) and third to Sigmund Freud (Smith, 1982). Intrigued by these findings and wondering whether Canadian practitioners would evince a similar high regard for Rogers, I conducted what was at the time the largest study of the theoretical orientations of Canadian psychologists and counsellors. My results indicated that for Canadian psychologists, the three most influential psychotherapists were Albert Ellis (cognitive-behavioural), Carl Rogers (client-centred), and Aaron Beck (cognitive) (Warner, 1991b). For Canadian counsellors, the ranking in my survey results was very similar – Rogers, Beck, and Ellis (Warner, 1991a).

One might expect that the results of these fifteen- and twenty-five-year-old studies would be outdated. Times have changed, and with increasing demands for accountability there has been more emphasis on evidence-based clinical models. Third parties responsible for costs now favour brief medical approaches, particularly psychopharmacological interventions. One might therefore expect the influence of Rogers and his client-centred, non-expert approach to be considerably diminished or passé with therapists. A more recent survey, "The Top Ten Most Influential Therapists of the Past Quarter-Century," however, found that Rogers ranked first[1] by a landslide (Cook, 2007). These recent findings support my continuing belief in the value of the client-centred approach and in the power of self-healing in the therapeutic process. If being listened to and the experience of being understood are necessary and sufficient healing conditions, as the client-centred approach maintains, then psychological recovery is primarily about self-healing – a notion consistent with the solution-focused approach.

The Importance of Understanding in Human Development

One of Carl Rogers's greatest scientific legacies was his research that first identified the three conditions for psychological growth and human development – empathic understanding, unconditional positive regard, and genuineness. When these "healing conditions" were embodied by the therapist, research indicated that clients tended to improve in therapy. The effectiveness of these healing conditions is not limited to professional treatment situations, but applies to all human interactions and relationships. The most powerful resources we have to offer others are our abilities to listen, to show that we care, and to be honest. Of the three healing conditions, the one that is most amenable to improvement either through training or life experience is empathic understanding or listening. One of the most frequently reported findings from surveys that ask clients to identify the most helpful aspects of their counselling or psychotherapy experience is that clients felt understood and accepted during meetings with their therapists. Empathy also plays a significant role in the healthcare field. Taking the time to elicit patient views and to demonstrate empathic understanding is central to patient-centred care. Furthermore, patient-centred care has increasingly been found to improve patient outcomes in medical practice (Rachlis, 2004).

When we are faced with upsetting situations or are suffering from psychological trauma, the experience of being heard and understood

---

1 The second and third places went to Aaron Beck (cognitive) and Salvador Minuchin (family systems), respectively.

produces a calming or "normalizing" effect by reducing personal isolation and increasing the sense of hope that things can be better. Our enhanced sense of optimism will often lead us to take a more active role in doing things that improve our situation. Regarding the role of optimism in helping us make changes, one particularly thorough study found that the single item that best predicted satisfaction with therapy was that "the counsellor encouraged me to believe that I could improve my situation" (Talley, 1992). This strong result (accounting for 68 per cent of the variance) surprised researchers because the treatment offered in this study was essentially insight-focused (psychoanalytic). Researchers in this study expected clients to choose a survey item dealing with "understanding their problems better" as the most important factor in their improvement.

Client and Counsellor Satisfaction: The Ryerson University Study

My interests in brief therapy and in understanding the factors that contribute to client satisfaction in treatment led me to undertake a new study at Ryerson University in 1996. The purpose of the study was to determine whether there was a relationship between client satisfaction and the number of counselling sessions attended. The clients in this study were students who sought personal counselling at a large urban Canadian university. I wanted to know specifically whether those clients who received the fewest sessions were satisfied with their counselling and whether they perceived their treatment as having been helpful with their problems. This study was important from an administrative viewpoint, as it raised resource-utilization issues. Could briefer therapy be as effective as longer-term therapy? The results of the Ryerson study indicated that there was no relationship between client satisfaction and length of treatment (Warner, 1996). Those clients who attended a smaller number of sessions (1–3) reported as much satisfaction with respect to their primary and secondary problems, and as much overall satisfaction with the counselling, as those who attended a larger number of sessions (4–20). Also, 75 per cent of the clients who had attended only one session for personal counselling (20 per cent of the sample) reported that they were satisfied with their treatment.

Counsellors in this study underestimated their clients' treatment gains with respect to both primary and secondary problems as compared with their clients' self-assessment of their gains. Counsellors perceived therapy to have been more helpful for those clients they had seen for more sessions. This was not consistent with the client reports. And counsellors were least satisfied with the counselling process for those clients whom they saw for fewer sessions. This again did not concur with their clients' experiences. These findings were consistent with research that showed that practitioners frequently underestimate the benefits of briefer treatments and tend to be more satisfied with longer-term treatment (Bloom, 1992; Steenbarger, 1994; Warner, 1996b).

Negative Human Interactions

One of the most dramatic illustrations of the lethal effects of intentionally increased negativity occurred at an American prisoner-of-war (POW) camp during the North Korean conflict. After the Korean War, 1000 American POWs from this camp were studied (Mayer, 1967). Incidences of physical abuse at the POW camp were very low. There was no barbed wire, no armed guard patrol, but none of the prisoners attempted escape. The North Koreans achieved their purpose by employing psychological warfare tactics. Mutual trust among the prisoners was diminished by rewarding the prisoners for snitching on each other (but the reported-on POWs were not punished). To ensure that emotional support was not received from home, the only communications the prisoners received from the outside world were negative or unpleasant letters (e.g., the wife giving up hope of the POW returning; the wife remarrying; notices of unpaid bills and bill-collector notices). All positive letters were withheld. Another North Korean war tactic required POWs to participate in small-group "therapy" sessions in which they were required to confess their shortcomings, including things they could have done but failed to do. Dwelling on and becoming obsessed with personal failures and shortcoming is characteristic of clinical depression. The "negative group-therapy" along with other North Korean emotionally isolating techniques was so effective that most of the POWs in Mayer's study appeared to be depressed.

The use of these tactics resulted in the most perversely effective psychological warfare on record. The North Koreans' technique of markedly diminishing emotional support and positive interpersonal experiences was so successful that the camp POW death rate was 38 per cent – the highest recorded in US military history. It was reported that half of these prisoners died without any medical causes: they had simply given up. This state of losing hope and giving up the will to live is called "mirasmus," but the prisoners referred to this state more simply as "give-up-itis." Even after the survivors were finally released to a Red Cross organization in Japan and given an opportunity to telephone home to let others know they were still alive, very few actually made calls (Mayer, 1967). This example of psychological warfare illustrates the dire consequences of the promotion of negative human interactions – the exact opposite of the promotion of well-being and the provision of healing conditions to which helping professionals are devoted. Psychologist Donald Clifton was so affected by the psychological devastation of the North Korean POW survivors that he devoted his career to the study of how positive therapeutic strategies promote psychological well-being. This approach later became known as "positive psychology."

My Research on Negative Experiences

I, too, have been interested in the effects of negative human interactions. In the late 1980s, I investigated the most devastating losses that humans experience – losses associated with illness, accident, and the death of loved ones. I also looked at more common negative experiences in which individuals felt misunderstood or mistreated by those who supposedly intended to be helpful – interpersonally hurtful social situations that occur in significant relationships at home, school, and work. I then investigated whether the passage of time would lessen the effects of the emotional hurts associated with these negative experiences.

Following the studies of an American psychologist, Branan (1972), I examined these questions from a Canadian perspective by first surveying university students. I asked about the single most negative experience in their lives. Negative experience was defined as "an experience that made your life worse or had a negative impact on your development" (Warner, 1990). I separated the written responses of students in this survey into two categories – experiences of illness, accident, or death (of someone close), and experiences that involved interactions with others. Of the students in this study, 86 per cent reported that their most negative life experiences involved interactions with other people – with teachers, family, and friends reported in that order. Only 14 per cent of the students reported their most negative experiences as illness, accident, or death experiences (Warner, 1990). The students were asked to write about their negative feelings resulting from these experiences. The most common theme described their feelings of not being understood or of being mistreated, particularly by authority figures (teachers and parents). My Canadian results were consistent with the findings reported by Branan.

Did these responses reflect the youth of the subjects – their unrealistic relationship expectations and their being, because of their young age, more easily hurt by others? Would the passage of time and ensuing maturity temper their perceptions and evaluations of the impact of interpersonally hurtful experiences that result from perceived misunderstanding and mistreatment? To address this question, I conducted a study of senior citizens. Given that these subjects were 45 years older (on average) than the students, it is not surprising that a much higher percentage of the subjects indicated that their most negative experiences involved illness, accident, and death. What was surprising to me, however, was that almost 50 per cent of these much older subjects still reported that their most negative life experiences involved interpersonal relations (Warner, 1989). I concluded that the impact of misunderstanding was still a significant factor in negative experience despite the passage of time and the acquisition of maturity. The importance of feeling understood is central to our well-being and to our overall human development.

The Medical Model of Psychology

For more than a century, psychology has emulated the medical model – maintaining that psychological problems are like medical disorders, with specific underlying pathologies that first need to be diagnosed and then treated by specific healing techniques that remedy deficits. Client improvement in treatment, according to this medical model, develops as a result of the application of psychological theories and techniques that help the client to understand his or her problem and its antecedents. This approach often involves the use of specialized skills associated with medical practice such as psychosocial history-taking, mental-status exams, differential diagnosis, and treatment planning.

The popularity of the medical model of healing emotional problems and mental illness is reflected by the fact that the largest-selling professional mental health publication of all time is the *Diagnostic and Statistical Manual* (DSM), published by the American Psychiatric Association. According to one survey, 70 per cent of workshops and seminars for mental health providers were focused on treatment according to DSM classifications (figure reported at a Duncan and Miller seminar, 2001).

Despite the popularity of this classification system, the DSM approach remains controversial. Here is what some critics have to say about it:

> Psychiatric diagnosis represents a flawed extension of the medical model ... Diagnosis is empirically bereft of both reliability and validity. It is worthless in terms of treatment planning and engenders harmful attributions by the labelled individual, his or her family, and the helping professionals. Finally, diagnosis changes like the tide, depending on the prevailing currents of politics and the gravitational pull of the marketplace. Diagnosis, however, persists. (Duncan & Miller, 2000, pp. 53–4)

Psychotropic Medications

Reliance on psychotropic medication is central to the medical model. Medication is often the first and only intervention that patients receive. The notion that depression and anxiety are primarily a result of biochemical imbalances in the brain is, according to an increasing number of critics, an unsubstantiated view enhanced by pharmaceutical advertising. The belief that there are chemical solutions to our psychological and social problems and that taking a pill a day keeps the depression (or anxiety state) away is, according to these critics, misguided and possibly a public disservice.

Further support for the above assertions is found in an investigation in the famous Treatment of Depression Collaborative Research program (McKay, Imel, & Wampold, 2006). Clients who received sugar pills from the top third most-effective psychiatrists achieved better outcomes than clients prescribed antidepressants from the bottom, least-effective psychiatrists. How to explain this? In a clever investigation that conducted minute-by-minute analysis of therapist–client interaction, Glassman and Grawe (2006) found that unsuccessful therapists focused on problems and neglected client strengths, while successful therapists focused on their clients' strengths from the start. And of course this is precisely what is done in the solution-focused approach.

Also critics of the medical model are supported by consistent empirical research findings that the most important factors contributing to effective counselling and psychotherapy are not medication, technique, or therapist, but are rather the client's contribution and the quality of the client–therapist relationship. These two (common) factors account for 70 per cent of client improvement (e.g., Duncan et al., 2009; Hubble et al., 1999; Wampold, 2001). If these findings are correct – that the healing force comes primarily from within the client and not from the therapeutic approach or the effects of medication – "then the whole of the medical model of assuming the necessity of different treatments for different disorders falls apart" (Bohart & Tallman, 1999, p. 11).

The Positive Psychology Movement

The study of psychological development using positive perspectives began about a half-century ago. Psychologist Donald Clifton was so deeply affected by the horrific effects of negative social engineering on American POWs in the Korean War that he began investigating whether positive reinforcement could be as effective in promoting the reverse – psychological well-being. His views are elegantly addressed in his last book, *How Full Is Your Bucket?* The book is organized around a simple metaphor of a dipper and a bucket, but is grounded in 50 years of research (Rath & Clifton, 2003). Clifton's pioneering work on strength-based approaches was recognized in 2002 by the American Psychological Association, which cited him as the "Grandfather of Positive Psychology" and the "Father of Strength Psychology." In the same year, Clifton was diagnosed with terminal cancer and completed this final book (co-authored with his grandson, Tom Rath) only a week before he died. I highly recommend the book for those who want to read a simple but practical book about positive psychology.

Dr Martin Seligman, distinguished psychologist and past president of the American Psychological Association, along with others, formally named this field "positive psychology" in 1998. Dr Seligman argues that psychology's forgotten mission is to build human strength. He explains this new direction in psychology as follows:

> Psychology is not just the study of weakness and damage, it is also the study of strength and virtue. Treatment is not just fixing what is broken, it is nurturing what is best within ourselves. (Seligman, 1998, p. 2)

He goes on to contend that the major psychological theories have changed to herald a new science of strength and resilience (Seligman, 2011). This new science, however, is at odds with the predominant problem-based helping model.

This idea of building buffering strengths as a curative move in therapy simply does not fit into a framework that believes each patient has a specific disorder, with a specific underlying pathology that will be relieved by a specific healing technique that remedies deficits. (Seligman, 2002, p. 23)

The development of positive psychology represents one of the most significant challenges to the medical model: it offers an alternative to the predominant emphasis on deficits and pathology (Seligman, 2011). Positive psychology is beginning to have profound impacts on our understanding of human flourishing, including wellness and longevity. And interest in this new field is spreading beyond academia. *Time* magazine published a 46-page special edition entitled "The New Science of Happiness" in 2005, and the *University of Toronto Magazine* recently published a cover story: "What Makes Us Happy: Science Offers Surprising New Answers" (Easton, 2005).

The Broaden-and-Build Theory of Positive Emotions

The importance of this "new science of strength and resilience" is illustrated by the research findings of Barbara Fredrickson of the University of Michigan. The *American Psychologist* published her ground-breaking study, "Positive Affect and the Complex Dynamics of Human Flourishing" (Fredrickson & Losada, 2005). Fredrickson has been studying human emotions for more than a decade. Although we have known for some time that people who are more positive in their outlook live longer and are happier, Fredrickson was interested in determining exactly *how* positive thinking and the experience of pleasant feelings contribute to happiness and longevity. Fredrickson has developed the "broaden-and-build" theory of positive emotions.

For many years, positive emotions were considered merely fleeting experiences with little evolutionary value for human survival other than temporary distraction. The study of negative emotions (e.g., anger, fear, sadness), by contrast, has attracted most of the research interest over the last half-century because the link to human survival is so obvious. Negative emotions were self-preserving for our ancestors as they prepared the body for specific action, such as fighting or flight. These actions have distinctive physiological autonomic activity associated with them. Studies have consistently found that stress and negative emotion, especially if prolonged and recurrent, can promote or exacerbate cardiovascular illness and other diseases. This helps explain psychology's focus on negative emotions.

Fredrickson's broaden-and-build theory asserts that positive emotions (e.g., joy, amusement, serenity, love) are also highly evolved psychological adaptations that increased our human ancestors' odds of survival and reproduction. The experience of positive emotion widens the array of thoughts and actions called forth (e.g., exploring and playing) and promotes cognitive and behavioural flexibility. A broadened mindset, the result of experiencing positive emotions, carries indirect and long-term adaptive value because broadening builds personal resources, such as social connections, coping strategies, and environmental knowledge. These important assets, in turn, produce well-being and enhance future health. Also of importance is the fact that positive emotions quell the autonomic arousal caused by negative emotions because they broaden attention, thinking, and behavioural repertoire.

> Because the broaden-and-build effects of positive affect accumulate and compound over time, positivity can transform individuals for the better, making them healthier, more socially integrated, knowledgeable, effective, and resilient.   (Fredrickson & Losada, 2005, p. 679)

To sum up, the benefits of positive affect (pleasant feelings and sentiments) are as follows:

- It widens scope of attention.
- It broadens behavioural repertoires.
- It increases intuition and creativity.
- It increases immune system functioning.
- In general, it promotes health and longevity.

Critical Positivity Ratio for Human Flourishing

Fredrickson and Losada (2005) argue that evidence from several independent studies shows that flourishing mental health within the general population and within marriages and business groups was associated with positivity ratios of above 2.9:1. Positivity ratio is defined as the ratio of positive to negative expressions of affect. The authors make the point that a high number of positive sentiments appear to be needed to overcome the "toxicity" of negative affect and to promote flourishing. With a non-clinical population, for example, flourishing mental health was measured by having subjects report the extent to which they felt any of several positive or negative emotions over a period of 28 days. The positive emotions were amusement, awe, compassion, contentment, gratitude, hope, interest, joy, love, pride, and sexual desire. The negative emotions were anger, contempt, disgust, embarrassment, fear, guilt, sadness, and shame. The subjects who scored the highest on various psychological tests – who had flourishing mental health – had mean positivity ratios above 2.9:1; those with optimal functioning had a ratio above 4:1. Subjects with normal or average functioning had positivity ratios of around 2.5:1. (Subjects with poor mental health had been screened out of this study.)

A study of clinically depressed patients revealed a positivity ratio of 0.5:1 before treatment. After treatment, those who had the most improvement (determined by clinical ratings and self-assessments) had mean positivity ratios of 4.3:1. Among those who showed average improvement or no improvement, the ratios were 2.3:1 and 0.7:1, respectively.

Regarding positivity ratios in marriage, reports on two decades of research by Gottman and Krokoff (1989) show that flourishing marriages had positivity ratios of at least 5:1, and unions identified as being headed for dissolution – languishing marriages at best – had mean positivity ratios of less than 1:1. With regard to positivity ratios in groups, Losada (1999) studied 60 management teams as they discussed their annual strategic business plans. From behind one-way mirrors, the researchers coded each of the speakers' utterances as being either positive (showing support, encouragement, or appreciation), or negative (showing disapproval, sarcasm, or cynicism). Those teams that had the highest positivity ratios were from organizations that showed uniformly high performance across three indicators: profitability, customer satisfaction, and employee evaluations by superiors, peers, and subordinates. Again the 2.9:1 ratio divided the teams whose performance was the highest – flourishing business teams – from those whose performance was languishing. The authors point out that the 2.9:1 ratio may seem absurdly precise, but that this bifurcation point is a mathematically derived construct that separates flourishing from languishing behaviour with remarkable consistency.

Can we become too positive? The evidence that the authors present shows that indeed there is an upper limit of "effective" positivity. When positivity ratios exceed 11:1 there is a disintegration of the complex dynamics of flourishing. I would suggest that when the number of positive statements is very high, the statements are not reality-based, and thus are seen as insincere and artificial. In summing up their ground-breaking positive psychology research, Fredrickson and Losada (2005) state:

> These data suggest that at three levels of analysis – for individuals, mar-riages, and business teams – flourishing is associated with positivity ratios above 2.9. Likewise, for individuals, marriages, and business teams that do not function so well – those that might be identified as languishing – positivity ratios fall below 2.9. (p. 684)

How the Broaden-and-Build Theory Supports Strength-Based Psychology

It follows from the broaden-and-build theory that enhancing positive emotions promotes well-being. The questions used by strength-based interviewers are directed at helping clients identify their personal strengths and resources. This process results in client empowerment that in turn enhances positive emotions. The evidence is persuasive that increasing positive emotions and experiences in our lives is likely to increase our happiness, well-being, health, and longevity. The focus of the next chapters of this manual will be on learning the skills to ask strength-based questions that increase positive emotions. Before moving on to the "how to" segment of this manual, let's consider the relationship of positive psychology and the solution-focused model.

Positive Psychology, Cognitive-Behaviour Therapy, and the Solution-Focused Model

Positive psychology has the potential to refocus mainstream psychology away from a deficit- or disease-based orientation. Its focus is client-centred and strength-based and it emphasizes the need to understand the positive side of human experience. Specifically, positive psychology maintains that identifying and building on our personal strengths leads to amelioration of distress and psychopathology and also facilitates our experience of living happy and fulfilling lives. How does the solution-focused model fit in with this definition of positive psychology? The purpose of strength-based interventions in general (and solution-focused questions in particular) is to help clients identify and build on their personal strengths. This process leads to empowerment, a critical component of living a happy and a fulfilling life.

Joseph and Linley (2006) define positive therapies as approaches that share the fundamental assumption that "clients have the solutions to their problems within themselves" (p. 14). These authors, coming from a client-centred background, argue that positive therapies share common principles, such as that clients are their own best experts and have the resources within themselves for personal development. These assumptions are precisely the same as the assumptions of the solution-focused model. Thus, the solution-focused model represents an application of positive psychology.

In terms of therapeutic methodology, solution-focused brief therapy (SFBT) shares a commonality with the cognitive-behaviour therapy (CBT) model. The interventions used in both SFBT and CBT focus on goal-directed behaviour, namely, the activities of goal setting and goal striving. While similar in this regard, SFBT and CBT differ in that the goal formation in SFBT lies within the realm of positive psychology – goals are strength-based, positive cognitions and behaviours – whereas in CBT, the goals target problematic or dysfunctional cognitions, behaviours, and emotions. This is understandable, since CBT is a conventional, deficit-oriented model. The difference between these two orientations is illustrated in the following example. When using CBT with addictions, the goals target the triggers that cause drug-consumption and relapse. When using SFBT with addictions, however, the goals relate to cognitions and behaviours associated with "exceptions" – those times when drugs are not consumed – and to relapse recovery factors, such as how the client managed to stop consuming drugs.

Coaching and the Solution-Focused Model

Coaching is becoming an increasingly popular service within the helping field. There are numerous coaching styles and methods, including the solution-focused model of coaching. Berg and Szabo's (2005) *Brief Coaching for Lasting Solutions* is an excellent book on coaching using a solution-focused orientation. But what exactly is coaching and how does it differ from therapy?

In 2003, the Australian Psychological Society defined coaching psychology. I approve of this definition because it uses a science-based approach rather than the more popular but not validated motivational approach. Here is that definition:

The systematic application of behavioural science to the enhancement of life experience, work performance, and well-being for individuals, groups and organizations who do not have clinically significant mental health issues or abnormal levels of distress. (APS, 2003)

The best study of science-based coaching that I am aware of was conducted by Australian investigators from the Universities of Sidney and Wollongong. This study by Green, Oades, and Grant (2006), entitled "Cognitive-Behavioural, Solution-Focused Life Coaching: Enhancing goal-striving, well-being, and hope," was published in the *Journal of Positive Psychology*. Its overall aim was to expand the limited empirical base that supports coaching psychology. The impressive positive results of the study should not be surprising to solution-focused practitioners: the relatively minimal treatment protocol – a 10-week, 15-hour total treatment, group life-coaching program – showed that participants made significant gains in goal striving and psychological well-being and were more hopeful, and these gains were sustained for six months. The initial group-treatment program results are impressive, as is the fact that subjects who were followed for six months (rare in research studies) maintained their progress. These study results speak to the efficacy of coaching psychology using a solution-focused approach.

The treatment protocol for the subjects who participated in the above-mentioned study was based on a solution-focused self-help book, *Coach Yourself: Make Real Changes in Your Life*, by Grant and Greene (2001). This is the best research-based self-help manual that I have come across. It utilizes a wide variety of client-friendly, scientifically tested tools and techniques. I highly recommend this book to anyone interested in coaching using a solution-focused approach, or to anyone wishing to make changes in his or her life. One of the above authors, Suzy Green, has written an excellent overview of life coaching (Green, 2012).

Microanalysis of Psychotherapy Communication

Up until now we have been discussing how "macro" constructs influence human development and psychotherapy. Recent process research studies by Drs Janet Bavelas, Dan McGee, and colleagues at the University of Victoria have added a ground-breaking "micro" dimension to our understanding of strength-based psychology. This research team examined what is explicitly as well as implicitly communicated in therapy sessions. Analysis of what is happening in the interview is important because we need to understand that when we are trying to be helpful, our seemingly neutral inquiries and comments are usually "loaded" with subtle presumptions that can have a profound influence on the people we are trying to help.

Bavelas, McGee, Phillips, and Routledge (2000) studied the moment-by-moment communication sequences in psychotherapy. They describe this micro-level examination of the interview dialogue as microanalysis – the close examination of what is actually said and implied by the therapist. The authors persuasively assert that all questions embed the interviewer's theoretical presuppositions and invite the client to co-construct a particular version of events or problems that reflects the therapist's theoretical orientation. In the traditional problem-based paradigm, for example, clients describe their problem, history, or feelings, and are assumed to have deficits (typically intra-psychic pathologies) that need to be treated by the therapist. The therapist is considered to be the expert on client problems and solutions and thus resolves the client's personal deficiency by providing the necessary diagnosis, insight, or instruction.

McGee (1999) and McGee, Del Vento, and Bavelas (2005) have illustrated how questions can be used as therapeutic interventions. The problem-based therapist often asks questions that embed presuppositions about pathology and the importance of the past. For example, as Wade (1997, 2000) pointed out, a traditional therapist might ask how the client "was affected by" the abuse. This type of question implies passivity – the client has a victim status with little control. But it can also be argued that victims often engage in "imaginative and judicious resistance," which, from a strength-based perspective, demands to be explored. In contrast, then, a strength-based practitioner might ask how the client "responded to" or "coped with" the abuse. This type of questioning implies clients have survival skills that helped them get through the ordeal.

All therapeutic conversations and helping interviews are unavoidably directive. The researchers eloquently illustrate this as follows:

> A question constrains the recipient to answer within a framework of presuppositions set by the question. In doing so, the answerer contributes to the perspective imposed by the question and accepts it as a shared perspective. If the question asks about the client's abilities and solutions, then the client can provide evidence of these from his or her life. If the question asks about problems and pathologies, then the client is likely to join in and provide evidence that co-constructs a different view of his or her life. (McGee, Del Vento, & Bavelas, 2005, p. 371)

Microanalysis and Solution-Focused Brief Therapy

When a solution-focused interviewer asks questions that are positive in orientation – about client strengths, resources, and hopes for the future – clients are invited to answer from a framework that accepts that these are an important part of their life experience. The client and interviewer will then work together to co-construct goals within this positive framework – a framework that presumes that the solution to the difficulty will emerge from these already existing strengths and resources. Here are several examples that illustrate how the interviewer's question presupposes that the client possesses strengths and resources:

CLIENT: I used to be promiscuous, but I'm not anymore.
THERAPIST: What made you decide to change from being promiscuous to not being promiscuous?

A microanalysis of this question reveals the following presuppositions:

• That the client made a conscious decision to change the behaviour, and
• That the client was the agent of the changed behaviour. (McGee et al., 2005)

The question is positive in orientation – it gives the client credit for the changed behaviour – and encourages the client to talk about the strengths and resources that allowed her to make this change. In contrast, familiar problem-focused questions, such as "When did you start being promiscuous?" encourage an exploration of the client's deficits – the opposite of the intention of strength-based inquiries.

Now let's look at how the process works with the use of de Shazer's familiar "miracle question":

If there was a miracle one night while you were sleeping and the problem that brought you here today was gone when you woke up, how would you know? What would be the first thing you would notice?

A microanalysis of this question reveals the following presuppositions:

• That the problem might conceivably disappear, and
• That if it did the client would notice specific observable events.

This question imposes a perspective that is both positive and future-oriented – that there is hope for a future when this problem is no longer an issue and that the client can create his or her preferred future.

Microanalysis of Empathic Responses

Empathic responses also embed important presuppositions. For example, an empathic response or formulation could emphasize the strength or the deficit component of a client's story. In the solution-focused model, interviewer empathic responses are positive, emphasize client strengths, and reflect the following presuppositions:

- Client statements contain some personal strength (or resource).
- Strengths are important and relevant to client goals.
- Exploring strengths is more important than understanding problems or deficits.
- Strengths provide the basis for constructing a solution to the client's problem.

The above presuppositions reflect the core beliefs of the SFBT model. Even though all positive therapies share a belief that clients are their own best experts (Joseph & Linley, 2006), these beliefs and the above presuppositions are not necessarily equally reflected in their interventions – questions and empathic responses or formulations.

A microanalysis study by Tomori and Bavelas (2007) underscores the above. When interviewers engage in dialogue with clients – even when they are not asking questions – there are nevertheless embedded presuppositions. This recent research also shows us that formulations used in client-centred interviews, despite the therapists' intentions to be empathic, were consistently negative in their orientation. Tomori and Bavelas compared the dialogue of SFBT (de Shazer and Berg) and client-centred (Rogers and Raskin) therapists using microanalysis. The differences that the researchers found between these two therapy orientations were, in one sense, what would be expected. The solution-focused interviewers used questions as well as formulations to communicate with their clients; the client-centred therapists used formulations almost exclusively. However, the researchers also found that whereas the solution-focused therapists' questions and formulations were primarily positive, those of the client-centred therapists (mainly formulations) were primarily negative, and rarely neutral or positive.

This type of microanalysis is of the utmost importance, especially for those learning interviewing skills. Our dialogue with clients – whether we are empathizing with difficulties, summarizing or clarifying what the client has said, or asking questions – is directive. The fact that we *intend* our remarks to emphasize client strengths, resources, and goals does not entitle us to assume that our dialogue will reflect our intentions. We need to take the utmost care when formulating our responses to clients to ensure that we actually say what we mean and that our dialogue reflects our beliefs and presuppositions. As Tomori and Bavelas state,

> It appears that the possibility of positive or negative input from the therapist is always present, regardless of case details, and it is the choice that determines what direction the therapy will go. (p. 13)

If the choice is to conduct a solution-focused interview, questions and formulations are required to be positive in orientation. When the interviewer meets this requirement, clients are invited to accept a framework that recognizes that they have the strengths and resources to find solutions to their difficulties.

This process research shows us that the dialogue of helping interviews always carries underlying assumptions. Because these assumptions can have a profound influence on our clients, it is important to examine our interviews at a micro level to ensure that our questions and formulations reflect our intentions.

Concluding Remarks

More than 40 years of empirical studies have consistently demonstrated that approximately 66 per cent of all clients benefit or "show improvement" in therapy regardless of treatment model (Bergin & Garfield, 1994). More recent meta-analyses indicate that the therapeutic benefits of all the different psychological approaches relate to four "common factors." Client factors – those labelled "strengths and resources" in SFBT – and the quality of the relationship between therapist and client account for 70 per cent of the variance (Duncan et al., 2009; Hubble et al., 1999; Wampold, 2001). The remaining factors – therapist model and client hopes or expectations – each account for 15 per cent.

SFBT, as a relatively new and not widely embraced model, was not included in these common-factor meta-analyses. The largest follow-up study of SFBT (De Jong & Berg, 2008) was conducted at the Brief Family Therapy Centre (BFTC) in Milwaukee – the home of solution-focused brief therapy. In this study of 275 hard-to-serve clients (57 per cent unemployed, 64 per cent visible minority), 70 per cent of clients reported improvement through therapy. These results compare favourably with the research previously quoted (that approximately 66 per cent of clients show improvement in therapy). The average number of therapy sessions clients attended in the SFBT study was three. This also compares favourably with the Bergin and Garfield (1994) study in which the average number of sessions attended was six.

In terms of the effectiveness of SFBT, my clinical judgment supports the conclusions outlined above and those of other investigators (e.g., Franklin et al., 2012; Gingerich & Eisengart, 2000; Greenberg, Ganshorn, & Danilkewich, 2001) that approximately 70 to 80 per cent of clients can be helped with the SFBT approach. Regardless of the accuracy of the above figures, Steve de Shazer, co-founder of SFBT, has made the important point that we have a professional responsibility to clients to begin therapy with the least invasive intervention. Clearly, a strength-based approach is the least intrusive psychotherapeutic intervention. The suggestion I make to SFBT students and workshop participants is that if the client is not showing improvement after the second or third session, one can always revert to the problem-solving model, or make a referral.

For the past 100 years, problem diagnoses have provided impetus for the major advances in psychotherapy. For this century, I predict the major advances in psychotherapy will emerge from the science of positive psychology (Seligman & Fowler, 2011). There is now sufficient evidence-based practice to support the efficacy of SFBT (Franklin et al., 2012) – a therapy that is arguably an effectie application of positive psychology.

PART TWO

The Tri-Phase Model for Learning
Solution-Focused Skills

Chapter Four

The Solution-Focused Approach

It is liberating and optimistic to believe that clients are in control of their future, regardless of what kind of past they have had.

Insoo Kim Berg

Solution-Focused Brief Therapy

The solution-focused brief therapy approach can be better understood by contrasting it with the predominant helping model. The central presupposition of the problem-solving paradigm is that lasting resolution requires exploration of the problem, either to promote insight and understanding or to alter the thought and behaviour processes associated with the problem. The necessity of exploring the problem and its causes is based on three assumptions: that psychosocial problems have a specific cause, that the cause can be identified, and that there is a connection between finding the cause and resolving the problem (Walter & Peller, 1992). These assumptions are challenged by solution-focused practitioners.

Pioneered by the work of Steve de Shazer (1985, 1988, 1991), Insoo Kim Berg (1994; Berg & Miller, 1992; Berg & Reuss, 1997), and their colleagues at the Brief Family Therapy Centre in Milwaukee, SFBT represents a paradigm shift in counselling and psychotherapy treatment. In the early 1980s, de Shazer and Berg began exploring a counterintuitive approach – that of questioning clients about the solutions to their problems. This was in stark contrast to the usual practice of exploring problems and their antecedents with clients. This new approach turned the psychotherapy process upside down. In SFBT, client strengths and goals are identified and explored, and this process facilitates the transition from problem-focused dialogue to solution talk. Although several counselling or psychotherapy approaches place emphasis on client strengths and resources, these are the *only* change "agents" used in SFBT. The central premise of SFBT – and the premise that differentiates it from conventional problem-focused therapy – is that constructing a solution to the client's difficulties is independent of the presenting problem or problems. Little or no attempt is made to address, directly remove, or reduce the problem (Johnson & Miller, 1994). The therapeutic discussions are centred on discovering what the client wants (goals), identifying existing solution behaviours (strengths, successes, and resources) and exploring the future – what will be different in the client's life when the problem is resolved or when the client is coping as well as possible. The goal of the solution-focused model is to promote change, not insight or understanding, and this is accomplished by providing an opportunity for the client to engage in what is called "the solution-building process."

Assumptions and Principles of the Solution-Focused Model

Accentuate the Positive

The principle of accentuating the positive is central to the solution-focused model and is at the core of all its strategies and questions. Focusing on the positive – what is wanted rather than what is wrong – and emphasizing strengths and resources results in client improvement and empowerment. A person's capacity to change is connected to his or her ability to see things differently (De Jong & Berg, 2008). Because of its primary emphasis on the positive or "what's already working," the solution-focused model is sometimes referred to as a competency- or strength-based approach.

Construct Positive Goals

Goals – what the client wants – provide direction for the solution-focused approach. When goals are articulated by clients – goals that are based on what is most important to them – there is enhanced hopefulness and motivation to change. Goals need to be expressed in small, behavioural, and positive terms. Negative goals – stopping or not doing something – are unproductive and need to be reframed. We do this by asking clients what they will be doing when the unwanted behaviour is no longer an issue. As long as clients can be helped to identify what they want, regardless of the nature of the problem or diagnosis, the solution-focused approach can be helpful (Sklare, 2005).

Assume a Non-Expert, Not-Knowing Posture

What propels this strength-based approach and facilitates clients' discovering their own solutions is the fact that all the interview questions are asked from a "non-expert" perspective. Carl Rogers, in his client-centred therapy, was the first to reject the "therapist as expert" notion derived from the medical model; de Shazer added a brilliant dimension that thrusts the client more quickly, though often hesitantly, into the expert role. De Shazer added a "not-knowing" posture (de Shazer, 1985) to Rogers's non-expert notion. Clients are considered to be experts on their lives – on what will "work" for them, and on what they want for their future. Solutions to problems need to come from clients: they have the resources needed to solve their problems. The practitioner's expertise is utilized in facilitating the solution-building process.

Use the Solution-Building Process

The solution-focused practitioner is not an expert on client problems and their resolution; rather, he or she has expertise in the solution-building process. The practitioner's role is that of a resource enhancer, a support system, and a consultant in the self-change process. The solution-building process is facilitated by the practitioner displaying an attitude of complimentary curiosity towards client strengths, resources, and future aspirations. The primary interventions of the solution-focused model are five strength-based questions (de Shazer, 1985; Berg, 1994) that empower clients to use their own strengths and resources to achieve their goals and find lasting solutions to their problems.

Comparison of Problem-Focused and Solution-Focused Interventions

In my experience with teaching the solution-focused model and solution-building skills, I have found that the term "strength-based" provides the model with a clear differentiation from problem-focused models. As one of my workshop participants, a psychoanalytic therapist, said, "I consider my work with clients no less concerned with finding the solution – I am equally solution-focused!" The difference, of course, is the process used to arrive at the solution. One either explores the problem and its antecedents (the problem-focused paradigm), or one utilizes the client's strengths and goals to build a solution. These differences in process are summarized in the following chart, which compares the questions of the problem-focused paradigm with those of the strength-based paradigm.

Comparison of Problem-Focused and Solution-Focused Questions

Example: The patient, Mrs Brown, complains about conflicts with her husband over his lack of understanding of her illness and her growing frustration with him.

Description	Problem-focused	Solution-focused
Questions that explore:	Probable cause, onset, duration, intensity, prior history, and other effects of the problem	Goals, strengths, successes, resources, and preferred future
Examples of possible questions:	*Can you tell me more about what happens during these arguments?*	*Can you tell me about the last time you were able to avoid an argument over a contentious issue?*
	How does it make you feel when your husband doesn't respond or help out around the house?	*What has helped – even a little – to get him to do more around the house?*
	How does your husband react when you tell him about how the illness is affecting you?	*In the future, when your husband better understands your illness, how will you be different toward him?*
	Given the extent of these conflicts, have you considered leaving him?	*Given the extent of these conflicts, what keeps you two together?*

It is important to understand that solution-focused, strength-based questions need to be placed in an "empathy" context; otherwise, they could appear cold or unsympathetic and possibly strain the client relationship. How these empathy responses are formulated and delivered to the client will be discussed in the next chapter. First, let's look at the kinds of client problems and situations to which SFBT has been applied.

Therapy Applications of SFBT

One of the most frequently asked questions from my students and workshop participants about this seemingly simplistic approach is "Does it work in very complex situations?" I recall my first experience teaching SFBT,[1] when one student said, "This isn't going to work with my kids – they have serious mental health problems!" This student was the director of a residential children's mental health centre where the children had an average of seven previous foster placements. I told him frankly I didn't know whether the approach would be helpful. Despite my lack of encouragement, the student completed the course. After the course, he contracted with me to be his supervisor for an independent study course for his master's degree. The topic related to introducing solution-focused training to his childcare-worker staff and to supervision issues. He later published his study results (Triantafillou, 1997) and went on to obtain his doctorate. His thesis examined the effects of training foster parents in solution-focused skills.

SFBT is now being applied widely in mental health care, addictions treatment, and the healthcare field generally (Franklin et al., 2012; Greene & Lee, 2011). More recent applications of the solution-focused approach are in non-clinical fields such as education, life and executive coaching, business and management, and the entire range of human services, including community development (Franklin et al., 2011).

Over the last decade, my practice has increasingly centred on the solution-focused treatment of stress, trauma, and post-traumatic stress disorder (PTSD). With reference to dealing with stress and the associated increased risks of violence and suicide, few environments equal what is to be found in prisons. This was vividly illustrated to me when I took a six-month contract to work in Millhaven Institution – a federal maximum-security prison near Kingston. My role involved inmate crisis management and conducting suicide-risk assessments. In solution-focused risk assessments the goal is to devote at least half of the interview time to identifying and exploring reasons for living. I recall one inmate's story of his attempted suicide by putting a loaded gun to his head and pulling the trigger. The weapon did not fire. When I asked him what he made of this, his reply was "I don't know," (and after a

---

1 This occurred in 1991, as I was just beginning to understand and practise the model myself.

long pause) "I guess it wasn't my time." My response was "Oh, really? Can you tell me some more about 'not your time'?" This question and the related inquiry for more details, referred to as "microquestioning," led to a 10- to 15-minute increasingly animated exploration of what he still wanted to do with his life. By the end of the 30-minute interview, he was less guarded, more engaged, and hopeful. The most persuasive and comprehensive description of the solution-focused risk-assessment approach is in the book *Hope in Action: Solution-Focused Conversations about Suicide,* by Heather Fiske (2008). I think that anyone who deals with high-risk individuals would benefit from the suggestions and implications for treatment discussed in this book.

Post-Traumatic Growth

Since 2009 my therapy practice has been primarily with traumatized soldiers at Canadian Forces Base Kingston. SFBT offers an important alternative to trauma-based treatment models that some clients find difficult to undergo. Certainly no single approach is effective with every client, but as Steve de Shazer, the co-founder of SFBT, used to say, we have an obligation to try the least invasive procedure first. Clearly the expectation of our surgeons is that they will try the least invasive procedure first. Should the standard of care be any different for other helping professionals? The solution-focused approach is less invasive because the discussions in the interviews target primarily the client's strengths, coping skills, and goals, and do not address directly the powerful negative emotions associated with traumatic memories. What was once called "shell shock" has now been labelled "Post-Traumatic Stress Disorder." It is typically associated with symptoms of persistent hyper-vigilance (including nightmares and sleep disorders), flashbacks (re-experiencing the trauma), avoidance of stimuli associated with the trauma, and numbing of general emotional responsiveness. Up until recently there were only three generally accepted outcomes of PTSD: death (usually as a result of alcohol and/or drugs), recovery with impairments, and full recovery (return to baseline functioning).

One of the most promising areas of treatment for PTSD is what has been labelled "post-traumatic growth" (PTG). It began with the work of researchers Tedeschi and Calhoun (1996), and the identification of five post-traumatic growth factors that reflect positive psychological changes experienced as a result of the struggle with major life crises or traumatic events (Tedeschi, 2011; Joseph & Linley, 2006). These five factors are assessed in the Post-Traumatic Growth Inventory (PTGI), as follows: appreciation of life, relating to others, personal strength, recognition of new possibilities, and spiritual change. Individuals who have experienced traumatic events report more positive life change than those who have been spared such catastrophic events (Tedeschi & Calhoun, 1996).[2] In addition to using the PTGI with soldiers, I have developed a simple one-page version, the Brief Post-Traumatic Growth Rating Scale – see appendix B for a description and how I use it with clients and workshop/seminar participants.

The strongest support for PTG in particular and positive psychology in general is the US Army's Comprehensive Soldier Fitness (CSF) program. The goal of the CSF, a positive psychology intervention, is to make psychological fitness in the US Army as important as physical fitness (Seligman & Fowler, 2011).

The CSF program, launched in late 2009, is the largest well-being intervention, military or civilian, ever undertaken. The founding of the CSF occurred when Martin Seligman was invited to the US Pentagon to present the positive psychology approach to the increasing levels of depression, anxiety, addiction, PTSD, and suicide among military personnel. After listening to Seligman's presentation one of the generals responded as follows: "Turning trauma into growth. This is a big idea, Dr Seligman," said General David Petraeus, "promoting more post-traumatic growth rather than just focusing on post-traumatic stress disorder, and approaching training through our soldiers' strengths rather than drilling their weaknesses out of them" (Seligman, 2011, p. 152). Of course, this is precisely the solution-focused approach to all problems.

An important part of the CSF program is the requirement that all soldiers take a course in PTG. Preliminary findings from the testing of over 800,000 soldiers indicate that as psychological fitness increases, PTSD symptoms decrease and healthcare costs decline (Seligman, 2011). A recent US Army report says, "There is now scientific evidence that Comprehensive Soldier Fitness improves the resilience and psychological health of soldiers" (US Army, 2012, executive summary).

In my work with traumatized soldiers, it is rare to have an interview where a client has not experienced at least some positive life change since returning from deployment. The two most common changes

---

2 The Post-Traumatic Growth Inventory is available online: see American Psychological Association (2009) in References.

I have noticed in the soldiers are increased appreciation of the value (and fragility) of life, and of the importance of family. When I ask soldiers what has helped them survive, the most common response is "My kids. They keep me going." Then I typically proceed to inquire about how the kids are important, and encourage the soldiers to explain, as concretely as they can, how thinking about the children made the difference, and enhanced the will to survive. One solution-focused author, Bannick (2014), states that SFBT can create "post-traumatic success" in PTSD clients. She argues that the nature of the SFBT approach encourages post-traumatic growth, and that growth is more than recovery to "baseline" functioning, but makes the individual stronger. In addition to offering individual SFBT to traumatized soldiers at Canadian Forces Base Kingston, we have started the first (to my knowledge) post-traumatic-growth treatment groups, with encouraging results. Also encouraging is the recent peer recognition reflected in the invitation I have received to make a presentation, "Promoting Post-Traumatic Growth," to the Canadian Military and Veterans Health Research Forum at Queen's University (Warner, 2012).

Solution-Building Conversations

The strategies and questions used in this approach can also be helpful in social, peer, and family situations. The solution-focused model is non-intrusive, because it does not encourage problem exploration or disclosure of personally sensitive or embarrassing issues. Asking a despondent friend, for example, questions related to the nature of his problem may require a level of self-disclosure that is uncomfortable. Asking the same friend solution-building questions, on the other hand – questions such as "What can I do to be helpful?" "Can you tell me about the times when things don't seem quite as dark?" or "How will things be different in the future when this problem is resolved?" – is at worst benign and at best respectful and helpful, particularly if undertaken in the context of empathic understanding. One doesn't need training as a psychologist or social worker to be able to use these strength-based questions effectively in conversations with important people in our lives.

I have observed the fact that students and workshop participants learn to use solution-building skills by practising in non-work-related situations. Students are often amazed at how helpful the strength-based approach is when talking to family, friends, and co-workers who are experiencing challenging life situations. Novices learning solution-building skills discover how to identify and handle situations in which the friend or family member just wants to be listened to and is not yet ready to do anything about the problem. A goal-oriented question (phase 2, discussed in chapter 6) such as "So what do you want to do about this?" in this situation is not helpful and often results in some kind of disapproving comment or gesture. Moving too quickly to goal-oriented questions in either social or professional situations is the most common error of the solution-building process. If I am complaining about something to a friend, and she asks a goal-oriented question such as "So what would you like to do about that situation to make it better?" before I am ready, I usually ignore the question, because it is not helpful.

Learning to use a strength-based approach with others also affects our ways of handling personal frustrations and the adversities of everyday life. Let me illustrate with a personal example. My wife, Janet, is the person I turn to first when I want some help or advice. I discuss with her what is bothering me, and after a few minutes leave and go back to my desk feeling better and being clearer about what I need to do. It took me a while to realize that the pattern of our discussions is solution-focused (though I had previously noticed how Janet was solution-focused with others, particularly her children). When I seek her advice, I might explain the problem and ask, "What do you think I should do?" Her pattern is usually to say something that shows empathy first (e.g., "I can see that that is a tough situation."), and then, often, to respond inquisitively with something like "What do *you* think you should do?" I clearly remember that my initial thought the first few times she did this was "But I left my desk and work and sought you out to get your opinion on this!" My second reaction, coming a split second later, was the urge to tell her my opinion and express my ideas – the contradiction didn't matter. After I state my view she will either agree with me or make other observations. What is most helpful to me is that she has validated my concern by being empathic and has asked for my opinion, which provides me with an opportunity to "think out loud" and to come up with my own solutions. Solution-focused thinking has become part of our relationship, and whenever one of us is upset by something, the other usually offers empathy followed by a strength-based response that is almost always helpful.

Development of the Tri-Phase Approach: Assessing Skills

When I first started teaching the solution-focused model in my graduate course at the University of Toronto, I introduced the principles and assumptions and then moved directly to the primary intervention tools – the five "driver" questions/interventions (see chapter 2) that drive solution building. I evaluated the students' skill development by comparing the number of solution-building versus problem-based interventions used by students with "clients" in peer-counselling interviews. (Students had the opportunity to be both "clients" and "interviewers" during the evaluative process.) By the end of the 36-hour course, most students would reach a skill level at which at least 50 per cent of their interview dialogue consisted of solution-building interventions. Although this meant that about half the interview time was still problem-focused, many of the "clients" reported that the experience (of being asked solution-building questions) was surprisingly helpful. Those who didn't find the experience helpful usually had interviewers who found it difficult to give up the "expert" role and suspend asking problem-based questions. Student "clients" were often able to make positive changes in their lives as a result of participating in the solution-building process – changes such as giving up smoking, losing weight, or improving a relationship.

This method of assessing skill development – by comparing the numbers of solution-building and problem-focused interventions – is now part of the final assessment for graduation from the Solution-Focused Counselling certificate program offered by the Faculty of Social Work at the University of Toronto. Demonstration of a substantial level of skill in this regard is also required for candidates pursuing specialist credentials offered by the Canadian Council of Professional Certification (see appendix B).

Tri-Phase Approach to Teaching Solution-Building Skills

After almost two decades of teaching the solution-focused model, I have developed an approach that provides a template on how to proceed in the solution-building interview. This teaching method improves student and workshop-participant skill development.

Students are encouraged to delay asking any of the five intervention questions (these belong to the strategy phase, discussed in chapter 7) until two other pre-conditions or phases are considered. Learning appears to be enhanced when the interview is conceptualized as having three separate but interactive phases – empathy, goal setting, and goal striving (I used to refer to the latter as the strategy phase). The first phase – empathy – involves establishing rapport and includes identifying client strengths. The second phase – the goals phase – is pursued by asking very specific, detailed, concrete questions about "what's wanted." Emphasizing empathy and goals at the outset of the interview seems to slow down the interview process, encourage better listening, and minimize the client experience of being "solution-forced."

Evaluating Solution-Focused Training

In 1998, I evaluated 64 psychiatric nurses and other healthcare professionals who had completed a 30-hour basic solution-focused skills course over a 10-week period. Ninety per cent reported that they had experienced increased job satisfaction associated with their new skills (Warner, 1998). After reviewing these results, I began to wonder whether it might be useful to target personal-development goals during workshop training. If participants were to "personally" experience solution-focused strategies during the training program, their motivation to use this approach with clients and their confidence about doing so should also improve. I first tried adding a personal-development component to the two-day solution-focused interviewing workshop with another group of healthcare professionals. The participants, 26 public-health nurses and home visiting staff, were asked to select a personal-development goal. These goals became the focus of the two small-group practice sessions and at least one instructor demonstration. Stress reduction, weight loss, increased fitness, dealing with difficult relatives, time management, and parenting issues were the personal-development goals selected by the participants. To assess whether the personal-development component was helpful or at least had the potential to be helpful, the post-workshop evaluation asked participants whether they believed that this approach could be used to help participants make desired self-help changes and improvements. All 26 participants answered "Yes," suggesting that targeting personal-development in small-group practice sessions was useful.[3] Another evaluation ques-

---

3 The personal-development component has now become standard practice in the solution-focused interviewing workshops. Participants are asked to select their goal and to do some preparation reading before attending.

tion asked whether the training had increased participants' confidence that they would be able to make personal-development changes in the future. Of the 26 participants, 24 indicated "Yes," and two selected "Not sure." The final question asked whether participants felt that they had personally benefited from the workshop. Again, 24 of the participants indicated "Yes," and two selected "Not sure." Comments such as the following ones also indicated increased confidence in using solution-focused interviewing to achieve personal-development goals:

> I have left this training feeling confident of my abilities to achieve my goals.
> Not sure I am confident enough with my skills yet, but confident that this is the model I'd use.
> My relationship with my teenage daughter is where I will make the effort to look for the positive and listen more.
> I tried it on my family – it worked. Good results!
> I believe that I have to be able to use this thinking (on myself) to be of optimal benefit to the client.
> Probably the most useful training session I've been involved with. I've learned a tool that will be helpful in all aspects of my life.
> Thank you, management, for supporting this.   (Warner, 2001)

Results of a Three-Month Follow-Up Study

The above evaluation was done immediately after training was completed. The results were encouraging, but we were also interested in knowing whether the positive effects of training would persist. A three-month follow-up was undertaken with 76 healthcare participants who had attended solution-focused interviewing workshops. Follow-up consisted of an evaluation report and focus-group discussions. Forty-seven questionnaires were returned (a 62 per cent return rate). The following is a summary of the evaluation report and focus-group discussions.

> After BSFI[4] training, 91.5 per cent of respondents found that they experienced an improvement in job satisfaction. Another 85.1 per cent found the training to be helpful in reducing work-related stress. Further, 93.2 per

---

4 Brief Solution-Focused Interviewing.

cent had found BSFI to be helpful in their personal lives. All respondents (100 per cent) noted that they had found the emphasis on strengths to be empowering for clients and said that BSFI had influenced their thinking and practice. Of those who responded, 95.7 per cent indicated that they found BSFI to be helpful in day-to-day work with clients, while 99.5 per cent found it to be helpful in their interactions with colleagues. Regarding encouraging clients to take responsibility for solution-building, 97.8 per cent had found that BSFI strategies were helpful. Finally, 62 per cent of respondents had used the miracle question. (Bowman, 2003, p. 2)

Recurring comments from staff members during focus-group discussions indicated that BSFI had been particularly helpful when working with multi-problem and high-risk clients. Staff members stated that BSFI was useful in both focusing appointments with clients and allowing for more effective team collaboration. A frequent response among staff members was that discharge planning had been greatly improved after BSFI training (Bowman, 2003).

Chapter Five

Empathy Phase: Establishing Rapport

To see the world from a perspective not our own.

Traditional

In this chapter, the reader will learn

- The components and techniques of effective listening skills
- A way to assess his or her listening skills
- How to identify (and compliment) client strengths and resources
- How to handle emotions and negative feelings in the interview

Effective Listening Skills: Components and Techniques

The experience of being listened to and feeling understood promotes our sense of being accepted and in some way validates our self-worth. However, one of the most underdeveloped interpersonal skills in our society is the ability to listen. Most people are much better talkers than they are listeners. The purpose of the empathy phase of the solution-building interview is to help the client feel understood. The other phases of the interview should not be undertaken until the empathy phase has been achieved. If the interviewer's empathy response is weak or inadequate, solution-building is likely to be less than optimally effective.

Ineffective Listening Responses: Offering Reassurance, Giving Advice, or Minimizing the Problem

Offering reassurance, giving advice, or minimizing the problem are common ways of responding when someone tells us about a problem.

These listening responses are ineffective; they seldom contribute to the feeling of being understood or validated. The individual may even wish that he or she had not said anything. These types of responses are also for the most part ineffective in terms of helping the person to resolve the problem. In order to be helpful, the interviewer must construct responses that acknowledge the situation or problem and indicate that he or she has "heard" the person. Saying something that validates or normalizes the difficulty enhances empathy and rapport.

Solution-Building Example: Steve's Job-Related Concerns

Let's take the client Steve, who says the following to a friend:

STEVE: I didn't sleep well last night thinking about my job promotion interview today. I just found out yesterday that a full panel of four will be present at the interview. My stomach is in knots, and I have just recovered from the flu. I'm wondering if I'd be better off calling in sick – I don't know if I can do my best today!

Common, but usually not helpful, responses:

Oh, it's not going to be that difficult. (*Minimizing the problem*)
I've had group interviews, and I know you'll be fine – they're not that tough. (*Offering reassurance*)
Just remember to take deep breaths before you begin. (*Advice giving*)
It really works – just try it. (*Trying to persuade*)

These responses are unlikely to make Steve believe that the friend understands how concerned he is about his interview. If Steve does feel a little better, it will be because he talked about the situation – not because of the empathy response.

Better response, demonstrating understanding:

It sounds like it's an important meeting for you and you're worried about it, particularly since you've just recovered from the flu.

This response is more likely to help Steve feel understood and taken seriously. Once Steve feels understood, there will be an opportunity to introduce phase 2 questions (about what, specifically, he wants to have happen) and phase 3 questions (about how he is going to achieve it), which are the topics of the next two chapters.

Now let's examine the case of a woman who visits her church pastor because of a marital crisis in her life. Martha is 35, has been married for ten years, and is the mother of two children.

Solution-Building Interview Example: Martha's Marital Concerns

MARTHA: My husband Bill told me last night – out of the blue – that he's had an affair with someone at the office. He says it only happened once – he doesn't want to lose me, says he feels terrible and will do anything to save our marriage. I called Mother this morning and she invited me to come and stay with her. I have to make some decisions – it's the kids I most worry about. I don't know what I'm going to do!

At this point, it might be helpful for the reader to consider the following responses and decide which of them the pastor could use to express empathy:

(a) What kind of husband and father has Bill been?
(b) Have you thought about seeing a marital counsellor?
(c) Aside from the understandable anger, how do you feel about Bill? Do you still love him?
(d) I understand why you are so upset and confused about what to do, when this has happened after all these years.

The first three responses ask questions that are problem-focused. Response (a) attempts to gather information about the state of Martha's marriage that would be important in problem-centred counselling, but in less-experienced hands could well add to Martha's emotional distress. The implied advice in response (b) may be appropriate, but is premature: Martha came to the church to get some immediate assistance, and this advice restricts further discussion that could provide an opportunity for her to find her own strengths and the solutions that are best for her (which may, admittedly, include seeking professional counselling). Response (c) encourages Martha to explore her feelings about her husband; this could easily intensify her emotional state and could add, at least initially, to her confusion and anger. The exploration of negative affect is the domain of the problem-centred professional counsellor. The exploration of feelings, whether in therapy, interviewing, or conversations, is not part of the solution-focused model. The solution-focused approach is directed instead at bringing about positive change, not insight or understanding of feelings.

Although all of these responses could turn out to be beneficial to Martha, the last one, (d), has the most potential to be immediately helpful because it is empathic; it conveys a real understanding of Martha's situation without giving suggestions about what she should do. Thus, it has the least risk of making things more difficult for her. This type of response in professional counselling is referred to as a "reflection" of emphatic understanding and is most likely to help Martha feel understood, which is the goal of the empathy phase. Once Martha feels understood – whether that takes one or thirty minutes will depend on how upset she feels and how much she needs to talk about the problem – the pastor can move into phase 2 and ask goal-related questions (e.g., "What do you need to do right now to best look after yourself?").

Effective Listening Techniques

Active Listening

Sometimes simply listening without interruption is the most effective way to help someone. Non-verbal body language (e.g., nodding and looking attentive) and an occasional minimal encourager such as "uh-huh" is all some people need and want. This type of listening is particularly important in cases where the client is grieving over some loss – our interruptions and words can be superfluous. In the case of Martha, silence might give her more time to think about and explore her options and would probably be more helpful than responses (a) through (c).

Handling silence is a difficult task for most new interviewers. We tend to become uncomfortable in social and interview situations when nothing is being said. When clients are silent during an interview, they are often thinking and working out how they will resolve their difficulties. Once clients feel comfortable, they are usually unaware of silence. An interviewer who jumps into silences too quickly runs the risk of interrupting this important reflective process. When novice counsellors tape their early interviews, they are often surprised at how much talking they do and at the lack of pauses in the interview. Most clients will benefit from a more carefully paced interview in which the interviewer allows lots of quiet time for reflection.

Repeating Words

Sometimes the interviewer's repeating of key words or phrases is all that is necessary to indicate to a client that he or she is fully understood. In Martha's case, saying her own words or phrases, such as "Out of the blue," "You talked to your mother," or "You're most worried about the kids" back to her can be helpful because it indicates that the interviewer has paid close attention to what she has been saying.

Summarizing

Being able to summarize even a small portion of what the client has said is reflective of a higher level of listening skill. In the case of Martha, a statement such as "So even though you're not sure what to do, you called and spoke with your mother" indicates that the interviewer has a good understanding of the situation. This is a particularly useful and potent technique when it is not obvious what the next step should be. The optimal choice for the interviewer is to simply summarize what he or she understands, and then observe carefully how the client responds.

Empathic Reflection

In empathic reflection the interviewer identifies and responds to both the content and the "affect" of the client's words. This is the most demanding of empathic listening responses, as it demands a high degree of careful listening and comprehension. This skill, however, can be improved upon with practice. If an interviewer inaccurately reflects content or affect, clients will usually clarify their meaning. When we are upset we often struggle to communicate what we feel or mean. An empathic reflective statement, even if it is not quite accurate, can help a client clarify experiences and meanings. This is the hallmark of an effective empathic reflection – the client elaborates and gives more details about the situation.

   Professional counsellor training incorporates learning to use the reflection technique because of its tremendous potential for affirmation and healing. The skill is central to client-centred therapy, in which the interviewer accurately reflects the content and feelings of the client's story. An accurate empathic reflection to Martha in the previous example might be "I can understand how you feel betrayed by what Bill did."

The interviewer reflects empathy

1 By paying full attention to what the client is saying and how the client is saying it;
2 By suspending temporarily the expression of point of view or judgment;
3 By imagining being in the client's "shoes" to see how that feels; and
4 By pausing, and taking a deep breath.

Assessing Interviewer Listening Skills: Mother–Daughter Dialogue Example

Reading the following dialogue between a mother and her daughter and then asking a close friend the questions that the mother uses may help the interviewer to assess his or her listening skills. The questions used here illustrate scaling and relationship solution-building interventions. These strategies are discussed in detail in chapter 7.

MOM: I've been reading this book about improving interpersonal skills and the author suggests that readers ask someone who knows them well some questions about listening skills. Would you help me? Is this a good time? (*Question 1*)

DAUGHTER: Yes, what's the question?

MOM: Of all the people you know and have had conversations with, who would you say is the best listener – the one with whom you feel most understood? (*Question 2*)

DAUGHTER: Oh, that's hard – I don't know – maybe Reverend Tom – when I went to him last year about that Bible problem, he seemed to really listen to me and understand how I was confused.

MOM: Who would you say is the person who has the worst listening skills? (*Question 3*)

DAUGHTER: Oh that's an even harder question. I don't know – I guess Uncle Fred – he just goes on and on, and you can't get a word in.

MOM: Okay, here's the hardest question: Using a scale of 1 to 10, where 1 represents the poorest listener you know, Uncle Fred, and 10 the best listener, Reverend Tom, what number would you give *me* on *my* listening skills? (*Question 4*)

DAUGHTER: Wow, that is hard! – I don't know – do you really want to know? Well, you're not as bad as Uncle Fred, but you do talk a lot – it runs in the family.

MOM: So what number would you give me?
DAUGHTER: Oh – probably a 5 or 6, but I talk a lot too.

Up to this point, we have been discussing empathic listening skills and rapport-building techniques that are central to all models of helping, including the solution-focused approach. What follows are the strategies that distinguish the solution-focused approach from most models.

Discovering Strengths and Resources – Focusing on the Positive

When we talk to someone we trust about something upsetting, we will begin to reveal not only what the problem is, but also our personal strengths and environmental resources, including what and who are important to us. When we are upset, we are unlikely to be aware of these personal strengths and resources; if we were, we would not be as troubled. Helping people see that they possess personal strengths and that they can draw on these strengths when they are facing trying and difficult situations helps foster a sense of hope for a better future. The process of helping clients identify their strengths is crucial to solution building.

A good solution-focused interviewer is able to reflect back to a client what he or she has heard and is able to identify and point out some strength or personal resource in what has been said or implied. Clients are encouraged to talk about their strengths – to see them as assets that will help them move towards their goals. Interviewers can identify client strengths from listening carefully to what clients say in their descriptions of problem situations. Interviewers will also listen carefully to what clients say about their personal resources, such as relationships with people, reputation in the community, or financial means. The most important resources and strengths are those that are most valued by the client. Listening for and commenting upon client strengths and resources when interviewing can be a challenge. Many of us have learned to pay more attention to "negatives" – mistakes, shortcomings, what is not working – and thus practise a deficit-focused approach to helping others. When we pay attention to "what's wrong," we often miss "what's working," and overlook the strengths and resources available to the client in the situation.

In the example outlined above, concerning Martha, who has marital difficulties, are any personal strengths and resources evident? Although we have only a printed transcript and are unable to see any of the non-verbal cues that would normally help the interviewer, several strengths can be identified. In spite of her personal pain, Martha talks about how important the welfare of her two children is. She is determined, despite her sense of betrayal, not to be driven by emotions or to act prematurely. She talks about carefully considering her options and the best interests of the children. Her relationship with her mother seems to be an important resource. This could be explored further. Even Bill might turn out to be a resource if Martha decides she wants to stay with him in that he is (apparently) repentant, wishes to try to make amends, and says he loves her.

Identifying and commenting on client strengths and resources, however, is only part of the challenge for the solution-focused interviewer. The next section addresses another important component of the interviewer's task.

The Power of Compliments and Positive Responding

Solution building requires that interviewers give compliments to their clients. Insoo Kim Berg, the co-founder of SFBT, stressed the importance of recognizing and complimenting people on their strengths. Giving a compliment signifies approval, admiration, or respect for something that is important to a client. This has the potential to enhance feelings of well-being and in turn to foster a sense of empowerment. Many of us have difficulty giving compliments. I often introduce the importance of compliments to my students by asking them which of the following best applies to their personal or professional lives:

1 They receive an overabundance of compliments – recognition from others that is more than is really necessary.
2 They receive just the right amount of recognition to keep them feeling motivated and appreciated.
3 They receive too few compliments and not enough recognition, and they definitely feel unappreciated.

The vast majority of my students respond that number 3 applies to them – they receive too few compliments. When we take the opportunity to give more compliments we not only make others feel more appreciated, but we also increase the likelihood that we, ourselves, will receive more compliments.

One of my homework assignments aimed at encouraging students to become more strength-based (and less focused on what's not working) asks students to look for an opportunity to compliment someone in their personal lives and to report back to the class about the reactions they receive. Students have reported many positive experiences. The following is an example. A single mother with a 15-year-old son told the class the following:

> I arrived home very tired after a long day. My son was preparing dinner, even though I had told him we would order in this evening because I knew I would be exhausted when I got home. The kitchen was a disaster area! There were pots and pans and food everywhere and he hadn't wiped up any spills. My first thought was, Oh no, I'm so tired, and now I'm going to have to do the clean-up after dinner. I wanted to tell him thank you for his efforts, but to once again remind him that if he wants to make dinner he has to learn to clean up as he goes along. Then I remembered the assignment and thought I would try it. I told him how thoughtful he was and that I appreciated him making supper for us. I didn't mention being bothered by the state of the kitchen. During dinner we had such a pleasant time, and afterward he insisted on helping me (unusual for him) with the dishes, during which time he opened up to me for the first time in ages. Before going to bed that night, he came to tell me how much he enjoyed our evening together, gave me a hug, and told me he loved me – something he hadn't done in a long time!

Gable, Reis, Impett, and Asher (2004) have identified three additional common types of responses we give to each other that can have a less desirable effect on our relationships. Take the situation, for example, of a wife arriving home from work and announcing (excitedly) to her partner, "When I was leaving the office today, my manager called me aside and said he was recommending me for the new district supervisor position." The following are typical responses (with the corresponding labels) used by the above-mentioned authors:

- That's wonderful news – you deserve that promotion! (*Active-constructive responding* with an enthusiastic compliment – an excellent solution-focused response)
- Does that mean you're going to have to work more overtime now? (*Active-destructive responding* – pointing out the potential downside)
- That's nice, dear. (*Passive-constructive responding* – a muted response)
- Well, my day was just exhausting – the air conditioner still isn't

fixed! (*Passive-destructive responding* – a response that shows absence of interest)

The importance of positive statements to our most meaningful relationships is underscored in the pioneering research of Gottman and Krokoff on marriage and divorce. In a novel study (Gottman & Krokoff, 1989), they recruited 700 newly married couples and videotaped them discussing an area of mild contention for 15 minutes. Ten years later, they conducted a follow-up study of the couples. They analysed the ratio of positive to negative comments in the discussions. They discovered that a ratio of five positive remarks to every one negative remark in the original dialogues predicted marriages that were flourishing ten years later. Additionally, they found that 94 per cent of those couples with the lowest ratios (one or more negatives to each positive comment) were either divorced or in the process of being divorced.

Research is also showing us that employee recognition, positive statements, and compliments have significant impact in the workplace. A Gallup poll found that 65 per cent of Americans reported receiving no recognition for good work in the past year, yet the number-one reason polled employees gave for leaving their jobs was that they did not feel appreciated (Rath & Clifton, 2004). Critics may argue that giving employees compliments and recognition has little impact on a business's bottom line. However, a larger Gallup poll that surveyed more than four million people on this topic found that employees who receive regular recognition and compliments

- Increase their individual productivity,
- Increase engagement among their colleagues,
- Are more likely to stay with the organization,
- Receive higher loyalty and satisfaction scores from their customers, and
- Have better safety records and fewer accidents on the job. (Rath & Clifton, 2004, p. 28)

Constructive Criticism and Giving Corrections

Focusing on the positive (strengths) and giving compliments does not make the solution-focused approach incompatible with giving constructive criticism and corrective comments. There are times when roles (e.g., supervision, coaching, parenting) require direct corrective comments – comments that focus on mistakes or what is not acceptable. Too often, however, the attempt to influence by pointing out what is incorrect, inadequate, or "wrong" is not helpful and does not encourage the person to improve. In fact, placing emphasis on what is wrong or incorrect usually has the opposite effect. The person will often feel less capable and less willing to change or improve. When all or most of the attention is on the error or "what's wrong," there is a tendency for the individual to react as if his or her personal worth or integrity is under attack.

So, how do we make critical comments effective? The tone, manner, and context (history) of a corrective comment is of vital importance. Depending on the relationship history, a husband saying, for example, "You bought a new hat" can either mean that he is pleased (he likes it) or that he is displeased (his wife is being frivolous again). The husband's delivery of the statement – his tone and manner of delivery – must be just right, and the statement must be made within a positive context, if he hopes to make the comment an effective motivator. In the end, the sole arbitrator of whether a corrective comment is helpful or not has to be the recipient. The motives or good intentions of the critic usually mean little to the recipient. And pointing out something the person already knows, such as "You really messed up on that project," "You are putting on weight," or "That's a failing grade" is almost always ineffective. Such comments usually lead the recipient to believe that the critic does not understand how difficult things really are. In addition, if a criticism is given before a compliment in conversation, the effect of the subsequent compliment can be minimized or negated. So an effective, constructive criticism relies on its context, on the tone and manner of its delivery, and on its placement after a compliment.

As noted previously, in Gottman and Krokoff's research, there was a critical ratio of 5:1 positive to negative statements that predicted flourishing marriages. A similar critical ratio exists when we look at giving compliments and corrective comments. My close friend Dr Frank Young, who is a sports psychologist, informed me that in working with elite athletes, if the coach does not provide at least three to four comments on strengths to every single correction (e.g., what's wrong or what needs improvement), the athlete's performance actually decreases. If elite athletes who demonstrate great competency need a high ratio of positive comments to corrections in order to improve their performance, it would seem logical that most of us will require at least as many positive comments in order for constructive criticism to be effective.

The importance of the ratio of positive to negative comments is also strongly supported by recent empirical evidence from positive psychology. In chapter 3, we saw that the critical ratio for flourishing personal mental health, flourishing marriages, and flourishing business groups is 2.9:1 or greater (positive to negative comments) with the optimum, for best functioning, being a ratio of 4:1 or greater.

Role of Emotions and Negative Feelings

The solution-focused model deals with emotions and negative feelings in a different manner from most other interviewing and counselling approaches. When I am working with experienced counsellors at professional-development workshops, I often make the point that in solution-focused practice, we ought to play down the use of the "F-word" in dialogue with our clients. After a few raised eyebrows, I go on to state that I am referring to the word "feelings." Many counsellors and helping professionals have been trained to ask their clients to reflect on their feelings. Such questions are counterproductive, however, to the solution-focused approach. The single exception occurs when the feelings are positive; then we explore these feeling deeply.

When clients express negative emotions and feelings, we acknowledge these feelings by being empathic. But we do not attempt either to minimize the importance of the feelings or to directly encourage further exploration of them. In other words, when a client is talking about upsetting experiences, we acknowledge the client's experience, but we do not ask questions or make comments that invite the client to further explore what is wrong. Clients will often go on and say more about their feelings and their problems, and that is fine. We continue to listen respectfully and be empathic, but we also begin to look for opportunities to introduce goal-oriented, solution-building questions (phase 2, the topic of the next chapter). It is important for the interviewer to understand that high-interest, complimentary responses tend to encourage the client to be expansive, whereas low-interest or minimizing responses tend to inhibit further talking or disclosure. High-interest responses in the solution-focused approach are used when the client is engaged in solution building or solution talk (e.g., discussions of strengths, resources, successes, goals, coping strategies). It is critical for solution-focused practitioners to be aware of and fine-tune this unique communication style. We empower our clients by *selectively reinforcing* them when they talk about their goals and their personal strengths and resources.

To summarize what the empathy phase of a solution-building interview might look like, let's go back to the case of Martha's marital difficulties:

MARTHA: My husband Bill told me last night – out of the blue – that he's had an affair with someone at the office. He says it only happened once – he doesn't want to lose me, says he feels terrible, and will do anything to save our marriage. I called Mother this morning and she invited me to come and stay with her. I have to make some decisions – it's the kids I most worry about. I don't know what I'm going to do!

PASTOR: I can see what a shock this has been and why you're feeling betrayed and confused. (*Empathic response*, but does not ask more about the difficulty)

MARTHA: Yes, because I thought we had a good marriage and both were happy – and somehow I do believe that he loves me, but how could he do this to me – after ten years of marriage and all that I've done …

(Martha goes on to talk more about the problem. After a few moments of respectful listening, the pastor responds.)

PASTOR: Okay, I hear how traumatic this is for you, but I want to say that I'm impressed that in spite of your pain you want to do the right thing, and that you haven't lost sight of your concern for your children, and doing what's best. (*Empathic response*, followed by a compliment and a comment on a client's strength – the welfare of her children is important.)

MARTHA: Children, family, and marriage are very important to me, but how can I ever trust him again?

PASTOR: Children and family are central to you, but so is trust if the marriage is going to work – tough question! (*Empathic response* – repeats client's words and summarizes the client's statement, but does not ask more about the client's problem.)

When the pastor engages Martha as illustrated above, Martha will likely feel that she is understood. The pastor can now begin the goal-setting phase of the solution-building process, which is the topic of the next chapter.

Chapter Six

Goal-Setting Phase: Discovering What's Wanted

No wind favours a ship without a destination.

Montaigne

In this chapter, the reader will learn

- The "key" skill of effective solution building.
- How to reframe "what's wrong" into "what's wanted."
- Goal development: the three characteristics of solution-focused goals.
- The kinds of change: classifying goals.

The Key Skill of Solution Building: Being Patient

Before we embark on the goal phase of the solution-building interview, it is important to reiterate that the empathy phase should first be achieved – the client must feel understood and a strong rapport between the client and the interviewer should exist. The most frequent error that my graduate students and workshop participants make is in moving too quickly into asking goal questions. If the interviewer has not adequately conveyed an understanding of the client's problem situation – the empathy phase has not been achieved – there is a strong likelihood that the interviewer and the client will have difficulty in defining goals and building a solution to the client's difficulties. Many experienced solution-focused practitioners will begin interviews by asking goal questions (e.g., "How will you know whether this meeting has been helpful to you?"), but when interviewers are learning the model, I recommend that they begin the interview with respectful listening and making an empathic response, and move on later to goal-oriented questioning.

How important is goal formulation to the solution-focused approach? If the client cannot define a clear goal, solution building is unlikely to occur. Goals provide the direction of the interview: as long as clients can be helped to identify what they want, regardless of the problem or diagnosis, solution building can be helpful (Sklare, 2005).

Giving the Client Time to Reflect on and Ponder over Questions

Solution-focused questions are thought-provoking and are therefore challenging and time-consuming to answer. If asked the question "How will you know, when you have finished reading this manual, whether your time has been well spent?" most readers would probably respond by saying, "I don't know." Solution-focused questions almost always elicit this type of response. "I don't know" is a perfectly understandable answer that often means only that the person has never thought about this question before. Answering solution-focused questions almost always requires reflective thought. The co-founder of SFBT, Steve de Shazer, put this dramatically by saying, "Ask the question and then get the hell out of the client's way!" (BFTC training session, 1990).

The power and effectiveness of solution-focused questions resides in clients having the time to process their answers. If a client feels comfortable, has good rapport with the interviewer, and is given lots of time, this important processing begins to happen – goals and solutions begin to emerge through the reflective thinking process. The solution-focused interviewer, therefore, must become comfortable with silence – the time clients are using to think, reflect, and begin to clarify what they want.

Responding to "I Don't Know"

1. MAINTAINING THE SOLUTION-FOCUSED MINDSET

(a) Before understanding what "I don't know" means in the solution-focused context, an interviewer will be thinking something like

The client doesn't know the answer, so I need to ask another question quickly!

(b) After learning solution-focused strategies, the interviewer thinks,

The client has never thought about this question before: I need to wait, be patient, and trust that the client really does have the ability to begin to build a solution to this problem.

2. DEVELOPING COMFORT WITH SILENCE

(a) Being patient: Remembering that the client needs "space" to think and reflect.

Giving the client space requires practice. Counting slowly to five can help. Waiting quietly for a client to begin responding is usually effective. If, however, at least five seconds have elapsed, interviewers might want to move on to one of the following strategies:

(b) Providing reassurance.

Example: This is a difficult question – take your time.

(c) Using a relationship-context question (discussed in the next chapter).

Example: How do you think your best friend/spouse/parent would answer this question?

(d) Asking the client to *pretend* to know.

Example: "Suppose you *did* know (the answer to the question). What would you say?" (Insoo Kim Berg used this strategy in a BFTC training session in 1992. In spite of the contradiction, asking this question often works.)

And then, ...

3. RESPONDING POSITIVELY TO ANY TENTATIVE REPLY

Example: Okay, you would be feeling better – that's good. And when you're feeling better, what would you be doing that you're not doing now?

Discovering Client Goals: Reframing "What's Wrong" into "What's Wanted"

Helping clients discover their goals is not as simple or straightforward as it might seem. In fact, this is probably the most challenging task of the solution-focused model. When we are upset or troubled by a situation, we are most often only aware of what we don't want (e.g., we don't want to be unhappy, or to have pain or distress, or to be abusing substances). Clients reply to most goal-oriented questions by telling us more about the problem – "what's wrong" or "what's not wanted." The skilled solution-focused interviewer will enlist the client's help to re-shape "what's wrong" into a positive and concrete form that begins the process of identifying a solution-focused goal.

The popular radio-talk-show psychologist Dr Joy Browne uses two effective strategies to help her callers make the best use of their very brief airtime. The first strategy happens before the on-air interview. A call screener asks callers, "What is your question for Dr Browne?" Thinking about the answer to this question requires callers to move beyond the problem (what is troubling them) and gets them to begin to think about goals – what outcomes they want to have from their brief conversation with Dr Browne. The second strategy employed by Dr Browne involves using the very same question on-air. When clients get bogged down in problem talk, she will interrupt and ask the caller, "So, what is your question for me?" This direct inquiry helps bring the caller back to talking about a goal – something Dr Browne can work with.

Dr Browne's strategy of asking clients to think about goals before the interview takes place is an effective solution-focused strategy. In addition to pre-interview telephone contact, printed material can be used effectively to this end. Some of the social service agencies I have provided training to have placed goal-oriented questions in the brochures they use to describe their services and mission statements. These questions centre on what clients want to have happen as a result of their interviews with the professional – questions such as "What would you like to have happen in your meeting with our staff?" "What would be helpful to you or your family?" or "What would you like to see happen as a result of your meeting with one of our staff members?" Thinking about these questions helps clients to prioritize their concerns and issues and to look at their personal resources. Therefore, their limited time with the professional is more effectively utilized. And ultimately, clients are often better satisfied with the service they receive.

There are a number of similar questions we ask in order to get clients to think beyond what is troubling them and to ponder what outcome is desired. The solution-focused interviewer is always, in effect, asking this question: "How can I be of help to you in this situation right now?" Any question that gets the client to think about what it is they actually want from the interview will be helpful. Because this is a counterintuitive mindset – to reflect on "what's wanted" rather than "what's wrong" – specific and persistent prompting from the solution-focused interviewer is usually required.

Preparing clients before their first interview and using the interview time most efficiently are the main topics of Brief Helping Interviews,[1] one of the most popular elective modules in the Solution-Focused Counselling Program offered at the University of Toronto. These topics are of relevance because most agencies have strict time-and-dollar limitations to their services, but at the same time wish to maximize client or customer satisfaction.

Goal Development

After clients respond to a goal-oriented question, the solution-focused interviewer needs to ask them to elaborate with further concrete details on their initial reply; for example, "What would it look like if …?" Persistent pursuit of goal clarity will give the interview direction and help discourage circular and problem-focused discussion. Goal development is enhanced when clients are helped to define what they want in small, behavioural, and positive terms (De Jong & Berg, 2008). At the beginning of this chapter, I suggested that I might ask a reader of this manual this question: "How will you know, when you have finished reading this manual, whether your time has been well spent?" I often begin my workshops by asking a similar question. If I wait for a few moments, someone will usually volunteer to answer. What follows is a typical example of how I engage the volunteer. Note the way in which microquestioning – questioning that elicits lots of details about what's wanted – helps facilitate goal development and goal clarity.

---

1 This two-day module at the University of Toronto has this course description: "The solution building skills to conduct single-session interviews and brief discussions of 5 to 20 minutes that clients find helpful in facilitating the 'next step' toward achieving their goals."

INSTRUCTOR: How will you know whether attending this workshop was a good use of your time – helpful to you?

VOLUNTEER: I will understand the model better.

INSTRUCTOR: Good (*a reinforcing response*), but how will understanding this model make a difference for you? (*a not-knowing question*)

VOLUNTEER: I'll be able to use it in my practice with my clients.

INSTRUCTOR: Okay, good (*Reinforcing again*),[2] but how will you be able to tell whether it's helpful to your clients? (*Another not-knowing question*)

VOLUNTEER: I'll see my clients solve their problems more quickly and get on with their lives.

INSTRUCTOR: Okay, but here's a really tough question – I wonder whether you can answer it. When you understand the model, are able to use it with your clients, and they reach their goals more quickly, what difference will that make for you, personally?

(Note: I would only ask this question of someone with whom I have strong rapport and who is very comfortable answering my questions in front of the class.)

VOLUNTEER: (*Pauses for several seconds.*) I don't know … (*Pauses for several seconds again.*) I guess I'll feel more comfortable – my clients will be working harder at finding solutions to their problems than I am. (*What the volunteer wants to have happen is beginning to emerge.*)

INSTRUCTOR: So, this is what you want to have happen, that your clients will be working harder to find solutions to their problems than you are? (*Clarifies that this is a goal.*)

VOLUNTEER: Yes.

INSTRUCTOR: And that would be very different from the way things are now? (*Clarifies that this is a new goal for the volunteer.*)

VOLUNTEER: Yes.

INSTRUCTOR: So, what's one small step you could take to make that happen? (*Begins to question how the volunteer will get there – entering the strategy phase.*)

Three Characteristics of Solution-Focused Goals

Well-formed solution-focused goals have three characteristics. First,

---

2 Both volunteers and clients need reassurance that they are answering the questions correctly; otherwise, the thinking process dries up.

goals need to be broken down into small steps. Clients are understandably impatient, and want a total solution right away. Asking about smaller and more manageable successive approximations of what they want will often be helpful and lead to less discouragement than tackling large goals. Similarly, with clients who present with a litany of problems, it can be helpful to say something like "Okay, I hear your concerns about (*Summarizes the list of problems to demonstrate that he or she has been listening carefully*), but I'd like to know which one of these concerns we should start with today."

Second, goals need to be expressed in behavioural terms – something that can be seen, something that will be happening. The goals of gaining understanding or insight, feeling happy, or becoming self-actualized are not behavioural and therefore are not conducive to solution building. These feeling-responses, however, need to be acknowledged. Then, solution-focused questioning about these feelings needs to be oriented in such a way that clients begin to formulate goals that are expressed in behavioural terms. Questions like "So when you are feeling happy, what will you be doing that you are not doing now?" or "What difference will your friends notice when you are feeling happy?" will begin to help the client focus on an acceptable goal.

Finally, goals need to be expressed in positive terms, "doing something," rather than in negative terms, "stopping something." Stopping drinking, stopping drug abuse, or losing weight are "negative" goals, and are therefore not acceptable solution-focused goals. The client may want these things, but the goal needs to be phrased in terms of what the client will be doing differently, or what difference it will make when any of the former difficulties are overcome. It is much easier to place something positive in our minds than it is to remove something negative. A question like "So, what will be different in your life when you stop drinking?" or "So, what difference will it make to you when you have lost that weight?" will help clients begin to visualize a positive, "doing something," solution-focused goal.

It is important to explore client goals, even if they appear to be unrealistic – to get details, including what difference the attainment of these goals will make in the client's life. Often this line of questioning will result in clients' modifying their goals to something that is more attainable. If this doesn't happen, the interviewer can respectfully ask about the likelihood of the client achieving the goal. This type of reality check frequently brings about more realistic goal clarification.

Asking "Not-Knowing" Questions

Development and clarification of goals can be facilitated by the practitioner adopting a "not-knowing" posture, by asking the client what needs to be different, or what he or she wants to do about the presenting problem. The interviewer does not pose as an expert on client difficulties and their resolution; rather, the interviewer frames questions that ask what the client thinks will help. Questions are asked in a positive and curious manner. After the client states a problem, for example, it can be helpful to respond, "So, you want to change that?" If the response is affirmative, then the interviewer can express interest and curiosity by asking, "How could you do that?" or "What would have to happen for that to come about?" As the interview progresses, goals can change frequently and the interviewer needs to check regularly with the client to clarify what is wanted. I have listed below a few more not-knowing, goal-phase questions that can help clarify what the client wants and how motivated he or she is to achieve the goal.

- Is this what you want to have happen?
- What can I do to help you with this?
- How will you know when things are better for you?
- How important is achieving this goal for you?

The last question directs clients to reflect on how motivated they are to work towards attaining their goal. This type of motivation or "assessment" question will either confirm that the goal is what is wanted or will indicate that another goal needs to be considered.

Kinds of Goals: Classifying Change

In the simplest terms, there really are only two kinds of change possible in any given situation – either we ourselves change, or the other person or the situation changes. Let's begin with the easier and much less frequent case – the situation in which the client understands, from the very beginning of the interview, that he or she cannot change others, and accepts responsibility for self-change. The client's goal will be defined in terms of his or her own behaviour. Asking one or more of the following questions will help a client "see" the goal more clearly and will enhance the client's commitment to the goal.

Self-Changing Interventions: Not-Knowing, Goal-Expanding Inquiries

- How will that change make things better for you?
- What will you have to do to make that happen?
- What is the first step towards that happening?
- What are some of the other implications that this change will have in your life?
- What will others notice is different about you when you reach that goal?
- What tells you that this change might just be possible?

Wanting the Other Person to Change

Frequently clients wish for someone or something else to change – for someone else to "fix" their difficulty. This way of thinking is understandable, as many clients feel personally disempowered and cannot see other options. Since some clients believe that others are truly responsible for their problems, it makes sense to them that others should solve their problems. The belief that others have the answers to our problems and the power to solve them stems from our early childhood experiences, when parents appeared to be omnipotent and capable of resolving our unhappiness and pain. The deep-seated belief that answers to the most important questions lie outside us has always been part of the human condition. In ancient Greece, for example, the oracles were consulted in attempts to draw on the wisdom of the gods to solve human problems. The solution-focused interviewer needs to be aware of and sensitive to a client's need to have others provide the answer or solve the problem. We need to be empathic and acknowledge these wishes in a respectful manner. Doing so will often result in clients beginning to take responsibility for their difficulties.

Here are some examples of client goals that reflect the wish for someone else to change. In interviews or discussions, clients will often express a goal such as "to get (my spouse) to stop nagging (or drinking)," "to get (my children) not to leave their rooms so messy," "to get (my parent) to not be so negative," "to get (the supervisor) to stop being so critical," or "to get (the teacher) to stop picking on my child (my friend)." As noted above, when a client says something about wanting someone else to change, it is critical to respond by being empathic and acknowledging their difficulty – saying something like "Yes, I can see

why it is so important to you for your husband to lose that 50 pounds."
After giving the client time to reply to the empathic comment, the interviewer should be prepared to ask questions that will be helpful for
clients who believe that there is no other solution to the problem except
for another person to change. Again, these questions are not likely to
be helpful unless good rapport has been established and the client feels
understood.

INTERVENTIONS TO HELP CLIENTS WHO WANT THE OTHER PERSON TO
CHANGE

For illustration purposes, let's take a situation where the client, Jane,
wants her husband, Gord, to change – to lose 75 pounds – because of a
serious medical condition. The interventions that could be directed to
this client fall into three categories:

(a) Questions that help Jane talk positively about Gord and see how
    she could support Gord's efforts to attain her goal for him:

• What leads you to believe that he can make this change – lose this
  weight? (*This asks Jane to think about Gord's strengths.*)
• Have you told him that? (*Asks her to think about how a compliment
  from her might help Gord to see his own strengths.*)
• What do you think you could do to help him make this change?
  (*Elicits details about how she could help Gord.*)

(b) Relationship questions that uncover Jane's perception of Gord's
    motivation to achieve her goal:

• Would Gord agree that it's as important to lose the weight as you
  believe? (*Is her goal important to Gord?*)
• Would he say he believes he can lose the weight? (*This could be a
  reality check for Jane.*)
• What would he say you can do to help him to begin to lose the
  weight? (*Directs Jane to think about what Gord wants from her.*)

(c) Outcome questions that help Jane see a future with success *or*
    failure:

Suppose Gord changes – loses the weight ...

- How will that make things better for you?
- How will you behave differently towards him?

Suppose Gord doesn't change – doesn't lose the weight …

- What will you do?
- How would you like to handle or cope with that situation?

The interviewer's use of one or more of the above questions with follow-up inquiries to elicit more details will help many clients to realize that they cannot change others and that they can only take responsibility for changing themselves. Once this realization comes about, there will be opportunities for the interviewer to introduce one or more of the previously discussed self-changing questions.

Frequency of Goal Questions in Solution-Building Interviews

Even though goal-oriented questions are extremely important in providing direction to the solution-focused interview, microanalyses of numerous solution-building interviews show us that interviewers actually ask relatively few goal-phase questions. The number of interventions used in the three different phases of a solution-focused interview will vary according to the nature of the client's problem and the skill of the interviewer. But analyses of solution-building interviews completed at the University of Toronto indicate consistently that fewer than 10 per cent of total interventions are goal-oriented. The remaining interventions are approximately equally divided between empathy- and strategy-phase questions. A microanalysis of the first session of the videotape "Irreconcilable Differences" (Berg, 1992) revealed that goal-phase questions accounted for only for 3 per cent, empathy-phase for 55 per cent, and strategy-phase for 42 per cent of Berg's 137 interventions or responses (Costello, 2003).

Discovering a Goal: Fred's Conflict with His Father

By now, it should be evident just how challenging it can be to help clients reframe "what's wrong" into a goal – "what's wanted." I keep in mind the following question as I listen to problem talk, and this question is a guiding principle of my practice: "What does the client want out of this situation?" Let's examine the following problem talk example:

FRED: Every time my father and I get together, he is so intolerant and right wing and even racist, we end up in a big fight. I get angry and the whole family is upset. I go home feeling discouraged and I get really down and it takes a long time to get over it.

In the above situation it is tempting to begin the interview by exploring what is happening, what is causing the difficulty – asking problem-related questions. The following questions are common in the problem-focused paradigm, but are avoided in solution building:

Problem-Focused Questions:

- How do the arguments start?
- Do you get angry in other situations?
- Have you and your dad always fought?
- How often do you end up arguing when you get together?
- What happens when you're feeling down?
- What's the family's role in these arguments?

In solution-focused interviewing, instead of the above mode of questioning, we explore what the client wants to be different. After giving an empathy-phase response such as "I can see how distressing this situation is and why you would want to improve it," we might then ask, "What, specifically, would you like to be different when you visit your father?" This typifies a curious, not-knowing response. I have illustrated below five different options the interviewer might use with Fred to help him clarify how he might want his visits with his father to be different. What is important to notice here is that a follow-up goal-oriented question can simply repeat or summarize the client's initial response in order to elicit in more detail what he or she wants to have happen.

Five Possible Goal-Outcome Questions for Fred:

- Do you want to be able to tolerate your dad better and not lose your temper?
- Do you want to be able to avoid spending time with your dad (for now), and not feel guilty?
- Do you want to be able to stand up to your dad better?
- Do you want your family to at least understand your situation better?

- Do you want to improve your relationship with your dad?

In the following illustration, Fred has indicated that he wants to improve his relationship with his dad. The interviewer has asked the last question listed above. Observe how a goal begins to emerge:

INTERVIEWER: You want to improve your relationship with your dad?
FRED: Yes – of course I'd like to have a better relationship with Dad, but he is so opinionated and difficult, I don't see how that's possible!
INTERVIEWER: But that's what you'd like? That's important to you?
FRED: Yes – it is, but I don't see how it's possible – you don't know my dad ...
   (*He goes on, and the interviewer interrupts*)
INTERVIEWER: But that's what you want because he is important to you?
FRED: (*Nods.*)
INTERVIEWER: Say some more about how important it is to you that you and your father have a better relationship.

Fred has admitted that he wants a better relationship with his father (although he is sceptical about it and we don't yet know if it is possible). The interviewer therefore undertakes the task of assessing Fred's motivation for achieving this goal. If Fred indicates high motivation for having a better relationship, the interviewer could then begin using the third-phase, goal-striving interventions, which we will explore in detail in the next chapter. If he is not motivated to achieve this goal, the interviewer will return to a goal-clarification response such as "So, I hear that at this point improving your relationship with your father isn't the most important thing" (*Empathic reflection*) or "So, what could we talk about now that would help you in this situation?"

Example: Martha's Marital Concerns

Now, let's return to the earlier case of Martha, who has marital problems, and look at how the pastor helps Martha clarify a goal.

PASTOR: I can understand how you feel betrayed by what Bill did. (*Empathy response*)
MARTHA: I thought we had a good marriage and sex life – that's why I feel so devastated. And now I find I'm overeating, drinking too much coffee, and not sleeping well. I'm just not looking after myself very well right now.

PASTOR: Yes, I can see Bill's actions are a total shock. (*Empathy response. The pastor pauses, then asks a goal question.*) So, would looking after yourself better help you right now?

MARTHA: I don't know. (*Pauses for several seconds.*) I just feel so lousy. My stomach is all in knots.

PASTOR: I can see that things are really tough for you now. (*Empathy response*) But what would it take for you to you feel a little better – not so lousy? What would help – even a little?

MARTHA: (*Pauses for several seconds.*) Well, it might help to get away this weekend (*Pauses.*) – without the kids.

PASTOR: It would help to get away this weekend without the kids? How would that be helpful? (*Not-knowing question*)

MARTHA: I need time to think and begin to sort out what I'm going to do.

PASTOR: How could you arrange to do that – get away for the weekend, and have time to think? (*Not-knowing question*)

MARTHA: Well – Mom invited me to visit her this weekend, but I didn't want to ask Bill to look after the kids – I didn't want to ask him for anything! But when I think about it, that's silly; it would give me time to think about this mess. And I could visit my best friend Jane – we are very close.

We can see that Martha is developing a goal – to visit and talk with either her mom or her best friend, Jane. Note how this goal began to develop after Martha was asked, "What would help – even a little?" Martha's goal of getting away to her parents' home for a weekend without the kids meets the three criteria of well-formed goals: it is small, behavioural, and positive – it is "doing something."

Example: Jack's Problem with Physics

Here is another example of how an interviewer can help a client develop a goal. A first-year engineering student, Jack, is facing midterm tests and becomes highly anxious. He telephones his family and says he wants to quit school and come home because he is having a "meltdown." His parents persuade him to talk first with his faculty adviser.

JACK: I can't take it any more – I studied until three this morning and when I tried to sleep I just kept thinking, "I'm in over my head!" I'm having so much trouble with physics, but I have two maths as well and my English course has so much reading I could spend all my time on just that one subject! I'm never going to graduate and become an engineer! Maybe I should have taken arts – I could maybe come back next year and try that.

ADVISER: Wow – I can see how stressed out you are about these exams! You're even thinking about giving up engineering! (*Empathic response*)

JACK: Well, that's what kept coming to me at five in the morning – I don't think I have the right stuff for engineering.

ADVISER: You don't think engineering is for you now?

JACK: No. (*Pauses.*) – Well, because of physics – if I could just be sure I could handle the physics.

ADVISER: It would make a difference, if you were more sure of handling the physics? (*Goal question*)

JACK: Yes – that would make a difference. (*Starting to think about the possibilities.*)

ADVISER: So what could help you have more confidence about physics? What would you have to do?

JACK: (*Pauses.*) Well, when you put it that way … I think seeing the prof and maybe getting some help – tutoring. But that prof seems so busy, and I'm afraid he wouldn't understand. But maybe I need to try to make an appointment anyway. My parents will be so disappointed if I don't at least try.

As we can see, Jack is starting to think about a goal. It would be helpful to talk to his physics professor. This leads us to the goal-striving (formally strategy) phase of the interview – what Jack has to do to achieve his solution(s). With some people, however, becoming clear about goal setting, and what they really want, is sufficient for them to arrive at a solution without the in-depth third-phase interventions. The latter provides the basis to conducting very brief helping conversations (10–20 minutes) and single counselling sessions (discussed later). The next chapter deals with how to move forward to the goal-striving phase.

Chapter Seven

Goal-Striving Phase: Building a Solution

The future exists in our anticipation of how it will be.

Cade and O'Hanlon

In this chapter, the reader will learn

- More about the five primary intervention questions – the "drivers" of the solution-focused model;
- Which primary intervention to begin with: choosing a past or future perspective;
- The role of microanalysis and microquestioning in advancing solution building; and
- The importance of end-of-interview feedback, and of assigning a next-step action plan.

The Five Primary Intervention Questions: The Drivers of Solution Building

The goal-striving phase can be conceived of as the phase during which clients become empowered to achieve their goals and find their solutions. Clients are empowered by the interviewer's skilled use of the "drivers" – the five primary interventions or questions of solution building. It is important to reiterate that if the client does not feel understood (i.e., the empathy phase is not achieved) or what the client really wants is not clear (i.e., the goal-setting phase is not clear), the interviewer's use of any of these interventions is not as likely to be helpful. The two most common obstacles to successful solution building are insufficient empathy and the absence of clear client goals. The following are the five primary intervention questions:

1. "Exception to the Problem" Questions: Discovering Competencies

Problems – no matter how distressing and pervasive – are never experienced all the time – 24 hours a day, 7 days a week. "Exception to the problem" questions inquire about the times when the problem or distressing situation is absent or affecting the client less (de Shazer, 1985). We then use follow-up questions to explore what is unusual about these times. The interviewer's careful observation and persistent questioning about these "exception" times uncovers client competencies and strengths that can be utilized to help resolve or better manage distressing situations. Here are some examples of exception questions:

- Can you tell me about the times when you are not experiencing your problem (or when is it less intense)?
- How were you different when you did not have the problem?
- When the problem did not happen, what was going on?
- What do you think are the things that contribute to you not experiencing the problem?

2. The Miracle and Other Outcome Questions: Exploring the Preferred Future

One of the most powerful techniques of the solution-focused model involves future-oriented outcome questions (de Shazer, 1985). We ask the client to imagine a future in which the problem situation – the problem that the client is talking about in the interview – is resolved. And then we ask questions about what difference having the problem resolved will make. Outcome questions can be divided into four types:

A. THE MIRACLE QUESTION

The miracle question (de Shazer, 1985) is the best known and most powerful outcome question. Essentially, it involves setting up a mild hypnotic imaginary state (i.e., suspension of disbelief), as it bypasses the client's logical, problem-solving thought processes. The client is asked to imagine how things will be different in the future once the problem is solved. It is the most complex solution-focused technique and it requires a slow, deliberate delivery, with frequent pauses that allow the client to enter in to this imaginary zone. Here is an example of the wording of the miracle question:

- When you go home and go to sleep tonight, suppose a miracle happens and the problem that has been troubling you is gone – just like that! When you wake up in the morning, how will you know (or what will the first clue be) that a miracle happened last night?

Exploring in minute detail the client's miracle picture often leads to dramatic results. The client will frequently become more relaxed, more hopeful, and even excited by the new possibilities being created.

B. ASSESSMENT QUESTIONS

- When our interview is over today, how will you know whether the session has been helpful to you?

Note: This is a version of the question for readers from the beginning of the Goal Setting chapter.

C. FIRST-STEP QUESTIONS

- When you leave here today and are on track to reaching your goal, what is one thing that you will be doing differently?

D. FAST-TRACK QUESTIONS

- When the problem is solved in the future, what will you be doing differently?

In situations where resolution of the problem is not possible, the question might be worded this way:

- When you are handling this situation as well as humanly possible, how will your life be better? What will you be doing that you are not doing now?

3. Scaling Questions: Measuring Progress or Motivation

Scaling questions ask clients to scale some variable related to their presenting concerns; for example, the degree of freedom from pain or distress, their willingness to follow through on tasks, their confidence, their hope for the future, or their motivation to change. On the scale, 1 could represent *the worst things have been* (when the problem, the pain, or the despair was at its worst), while 10 represents when the problem is resolved or the goal is achieved. Alternatively, 1 could represent very low motivation to reach the goal, while 10 represents maximum motivation. Here are some examples of scaling questions:

- On a scale of 1 to 10, where 1 is the most stressed you have been at work, and 10 is where you are satisfied with the way you are handling the stresses of the job, what number best represents where you are now?
- How motivated are you to improve your grades? If 1 means that grades are not a high priority to you right now, and 10 means that getting higher grades is your highest priority and you are ready right now to work your hardest to improve your grades, what number would you assign yourself?

After clients mention a specific number, two further questions should be asked that will increase the effectiveness of the scaling question:

- How did you get to that number? (*Uncovers client strengths and competencies.*)
- What would have to happen for you to move up one-half-point on that scale? (*Helps clients determine what a small improvement would look like.*)

4. Relationship Questions: Seeking the Opinions of Others

The relationship question (Berg, 1994) is a very useful technique that requires clients to step outside themselves and view their behaviour from someone else's perspective. The relationship question is particularly helpful when the issue or problem involves another person. Here are some examples of the relationship question:

- What would your manager say you could do to begin to convince him that you are up to the new job?
- Knowing your parents as well as you do, what would they say they need to see from you before they would consider taking you back into the house?
- What do you think your best friend sees in you to inspire such confidence in your abilities?

- Would your child say that it helps him when you work with him on his homework?

5. Coping Questions: Survival Skills

When clients experience trauma or major setbacks, or are discouraged about their progress, it is usually helpful to ask coping questions. The aim of coping questions is to help the client reframe the situation and gain a more positive perspective. Such questions lead clients to recognize the resources and strengths they are already using in the difficult situation. In order to make coping questions effective, it is absolutely essential that the interviewer preface them with an empathic statement (*Phase 1*). We acknowledge the (perceived) dire position before we ask anything about how the client manages to cope or keep trying.

Once clients describe how they manage to cope, the interviewer can compliment them on their strengths and can then ask what it would take to continue doing what is working for them. The coping question is an excellent solution-building strategy, as it encourages the client to talk about strengths and resources rather than deficits and problems. If the client is asked about the worst day he has ever experienced on the job, for example, this would be encouraging talk about problems. On the other hand, if the client were asked how he or she coped with the worst day ever on the job, the discussion would likely result in solution building – the uncovering of the actions and thoughts that made surviving that difficult time possible.

Here are some examples of coping questions:

- How do you cope with life in spite of all the difficulties you are experiencing?
- What is one thing that keeps you going?
- What would it take for you to continue doing what has gotten you through this so far?

How to Begin: Choosing the Exception (Past) or the Outcome (Future) Perspective

Novices learning the solution-focused model often have difficulties when they get to the goal-striving phase of the interview. Not only must they decide which of the five primary intervention questions should be used to begin the phase, but they also have to decide what other questions should be used to follow up their initial intervention.

Conceptualizing goal-striving-phase questions as directing the client to think about either the past or the future can be helpful. Exception questions ask the client about the past – about previous times when the difficulty was not so troublesome. Outcome questions ask clients about the future – about a time when the difficulty will be resolved, or the client will be coping as well as possible. The interviewer has a choice about which time direction should be used to facilitate solution-building talk. Whichever direction seems more appropriate should be used first. If it is not clear which direction is the more appropriate, the novice can always begin the goal-striving phase with a question about the past – an exception question – and if this is not successful, can then employ a question about the future – an outcome question.

Scaling, Relationship, and Outcome Questions: Broaden and Build

The remaining three primary intervention questions – scaling, relationship, and coping questions – can be subsequently employed as supporting tools to broaden and build on the solution talk that emerges when the client begins responding to exception or outcome questions. Let's return to the case of Fred to illustrate past- and future-oriented interventions along with corresponding broadening and building questions. You may recall from the last dialogue that Fred came up with the goal of having a better relationship with his father. The table below compares the goal-striving-phase options of using questions from the past (exceptions) or the future (outcomes) perspective. Use of the other three types of questions – scaling, relationship, and coping – to broaden and build on the emerging goal is illustrated for both past and future orientations.

Comparison of Exception (Past) and Outcome (Future) Questions

Client goal: To improve his relationship with his father. The following questions illustrate the wide variety of options the interviewer can use to encourage solution talk.

Past	Future
Exception question	*Outcome question*
Can you tell me about the last time you and your father got along better?	In the future, when you and your father are getting along better, what will you be doing with him that you are not doing now?

Scaling question
On a scale of 1 to 10, where 1 represents when you and your father didn't get along at all, and 10 represents the best your relationship has been, what number would you be at now?

Scaling question
How motivated are you to improve your relationship with your father? On a scale of 1 to 10, where 1 indicates you are not yet prepared to do anything, and 10 that you are really motivated to do whatever it takes to make the relationship better, what number are you at now?

Relationship question
What would your father say he liked best about you when you were getting along better?

Relationship question
In the future, when you are getting along better with your father, what will he notice is different about how you treat him?

Coping question
In spite of the stresses and conflict with your father, how have you managed to cope with him as well as you have?

Coping question
In the future, when you have a better relationship with your father, if he makes a racist remark, how will you handle it?

A brief compilation of the most common questions used in solution building, divided according to the interview phases, is included as appendix A. Students and workshop participants have stated that taking a single-page copy of this compilation (or a modified version of it) into their interviews has been helpful when they are learning the skills.

Microanalysis: Improving Solution-Building Questions

The goal of solution-focused interviewing is to ask questions that lead to clients building their own solutions. But not all positive, strength-based questions are equal. To illustrate this, consider an example from McGee (1999) in which the client makes the following statement: "I used to take a lot of drugs, but I don't anymore." The problem-focused interviewer would ask questions related to the drug-taking behaviour, using responses such as "You took drugs?" or "You're still taking *some* drugs?" The presupposition is that the client's experience with drugs is what is most important to the interviewer.

In contrast, the solution-focused interviewer is most interested in the client's strengths and competencies, and will thus focus on the fact that the client doesn't take drugs anymore. The solution-focused interviewer might therefore ask, "How did it happen – that you gave up drugs?" This is an acceptable solution-focused response; however, it might be interpreted as suggesting that the credit for the change could be related to external factors. A better intervention would be "How did you do it – give up drugs"? The underlying assumption here is that the credit for the change lies with the client and it invites the client to look for evidence to support this view. The best solution-building intervention would be, "What made you decide to give up drugs"? This question presupposes that the client made a conscious decision to give up using drugs. The client is invited to talk about the personal strengths he used to change his behaviour. When we reflect on decisions related to important issues in our lives, we often become more aware of our personal belief systems – and when our decisions reflect our core values, our commitment to making and maintaining change is high.

Microquestioning: Uncovering the Details

As practitioners become more proficient at asking strength-based questions, they are able to conduct interviews that are almost totally solution-focused, with few or no problem-focused questions. What distinguishes the advanced practitioners, however, is the number of microquestions they ask about each client strength or positive behaviour they uncover, before they move on to ask questions about other themes. The process of microquestioning broadens clients' understanding of each of their strengths and resources and in the process enhances their empowerment and motivation to attain their goals.

When a client is talking about a problem situation and refers to a particular cognitive or behavioural response that appears to represent a change or improvement, the advanced practitioner can utilize a multitude of different options. For example, a client who has been struggling with a weight-management problem might mention that he went to a buffet dinner and didn't go back for second helpings. The practitioner's first response would be to summarize the behaviour: "You went to a buffet dinner and didn't go back for seconds!" Then the practitioner would add, using a curious, complimentary tone: "You were able to do that?" An interviewer using microquestioning techniques would then utilize a very important follow-up inquiry that would ask if this behaviour is unusual for the client. If the behaviour is unusual, the interviewer would then ask more questions about how the client succeeded in not having seconds. If, on the other hand, this behaviour occurs frequently, then it probably is not worth pursuing. The interviewer is looking for a behaviour that is both unusual and positive, an exception, because a praiseworthy single step in the right direction could, if properly recognized and rewarded, lead to sustained behaviour change. If the client is almost always able to resist second trips to the buffet, the interviewer would move on to ask a question on another topic.

The following are examples of microquestions that could be directed to the above-mentioned client if he claimed that not going up for seconds was exceptional behaviour for him:

1 You did that – you were able to go to a buffet dinner and not get second helpings?
2 Is it unusual for you to be able to do that?
3 How did you do it – was it hard?
4 Did your wife notice it – did she say anything?
5 Is that something you want to be able to do again?
6 How are you going to do it again?
7 Do you think it's possible that this could be the beginning of an important change for you?
8 What would help you do it again?
9 Can you summarize what you learned from this experience that will be helpful the next time?

Here is another example of what microquestioning would look like. In this case, an adolescent who has been having a lot of conflict with his mother (frequent loud arguments) has expressed a desire to improve his home situation. The teenager mentions that he and his mother had arguments for three days in a row last week.

1 Do I understand that you went for 4 days without fighting with your mom last week?
2 Is it unusual for you and your mom to go that long without an argument?
3 Would your mom agree that this was unusual?
4 How did you manage to do that?
5 What were things like for you on those days that you didn't fight?
6 How would your mom say you were different on those days?
7 Is that something you want to do more of?
8 How are you going to do that again?
9 What is going to help you do that again?

End-of-Interview Break and Next-Step Action Plan

It is not uncommon for the solution-building interviewer to take a "break" close to the end of the session. The practitioner will often leave the office or interview room for a few minutes and will review what happened in the interview and formulate feedback for the client that will include a task assignment. The feedback portion of the interview consists of three components: (1) compliments given to the client (usually on strengths), (2) a bridging statement, which is a rationale for the task assignment, and (3) the task assignment itself (De Jong & Berg, 2008). The task assignment is developed from the interview discussion and is given as a suggestion rather than an instruction. The client should be asked whether completing the task would be helpful. If the client replies "Yes," that carrying out the task could be helpful, the interviewer can follow up by asking the client for details about how the task might be helpful. This usually increases commitment. If the client says "No," or in some other way communicates low interest in carrying out the task, the interviewer can ask what the client thinks would be helpful. I prefer to call the task assignment the "next-step action plan" – this frames the task in an action-oriented context. Next-step action plans work best with clients who are motivated to do something as a result of having clear goals emerge from the goal phase of the interview.

There will be clients, however, who by the end of the interview will still be unready to take any action with regard to their problems. In these situations, it is better if the task assignment is an "observational" one. For example, the task might be phrased in one of the following ways:

- It sounds like you need to do some more thinking about how you want to handle this situation.
- Could you pay attention to when things are going better between the two of you – and what you both are doing to make it better at those times?

Three Types of Interview Breaks

Experience has shown that the formulation and delivery of feedback and next-step action plans are more effective if the interviewer makes use of a "break." There are three different break options available to the interviewer:

1. LEAVING THE INTERVIEW LOCATION

Towards the end of the session, the interviewer should introduce the idea of the break to the client. Here is an example:

- Okay, I have a pretty good idea of your situation now. Is there anything else you think I should know before I take a few minutes to think about what you've told me, and come back and give you some feedback? Would that be okay?

At my workplace, walking out to the reception area to pick up the appointment book to arrange for the next session provided me an opportunity to formulate the feedback and consider a task. The public-health nurses and home visitors with whom I have consulted tell me that when visiting clients in their homes, they might go out to the car or to the washroom to take the break, and that this works well. This type of break – where the interviewer actually leaves the interview location for a few moments – has the strongest impact on the client, and is highly recommended.

There are, however, situations in which the option of leaving the interview location is not practical. If there is time, the following type of break can be used in these situations:

2. TAKING A MINUTE TO REVIEW NOTES

Towards the end of the session, the interviewer would begin by saying something like

- Okay, I have a pretty good idea of your situation. Now what I would like to do is take a minute and review my notes and then give you some feedback. Would that be okay?

The interviewer would then turn slightly away from the client and review the interview notes for a minute or so.
Finally, when pressed for time or conducting a very short interview, reviewing of notes can be skipped and the interviewer can move directly into giving feedback. It is still very helpful, however, to convey the idea that the interview process is changing and coming to an end. This can be done through the use of a transition point – a verbal indication that the flow of the interview process is about to change.

3. INTRODUCING A TRANSITION POINT

The interviewer might introduce the transition point by taking a deep breath and saying something like

- Okay, our time is just about up. Is there anything else you want to tell me before I give you some feedback?

Rationale for Using a Break

Most practitioners are not used to taking a break in their interviews. I strongly recommend, however, that interviewers make use of a break or establish a transition point before introducing the client feedback and next-step action-plan segments of the interview. The break will

- Provide a pause for reflection for both interviewer and client;
- Increase the client's anticipation of and receptivity to receiving the compliments, and consequently will help the client feel better about him- or herself;
- Increase the likelihood of the client following through on the task – doing something to improve his or her situation; and
- Ensure that the interviewer is prepared to offer helpful feedback to the client; clients always appreciate hearing good things about themselves.

Delivery of Feedback and Next-Step Action Plans

Here are some suggestions about delivering feedback and proposing the next-step action plan after taking the break:

- Begin the feedback portion by summarizing the client's situation and goals.
- Give compliments on the client's strengths and anything else you appreciate about him or her.
- Suggest a possible next-step action plan that arises out of what the client says he or she wants to have happen.
- Observe the client's reaction, and if it is not enthusiastic, drop that suggestion and ask the client for his or her ideas.
- If the reaction is positive, ask how carrying out the suggested next step might be helpful to the client; ask for details.

- End the interview by summarizing the action plan the client has agreed to complete before the next meeting.

Now let's see how strategy-phase questions might be used with our client Fred, who has a conflict with his father. We will pick up from the point in the last chapter where Fred has been asked a goal-phase question.

Example: Fred's Conflict with His Father

FRED: Well, yes – I guess I would like to have a better relationship with Dad, but he is so opinionated and difficult!

INTERVIEWER: But that's what you would like? That is important to you? (*Fred nods.*) Would that be something useful to get out of our discussion today or do you have something else in mind? (*Clarifies the goal.*)

FRED: No – if you could help me get my father to understand that racism is wrong, and ...

INTERVIEWER: (*Interrupts.*) I agree that it's wrong and I hear how upsetting it is to you, but I can't change anyone any more than you can – and from what you've said, what you've tried to do with your father hasn't worked – right? (*Fred nods.*) So, I would like to move on and ask you another question, if that would be okay. On a scale of 1 to 10, where 1 represents that while the relationship with your father isn't great, you can live with it for now – you're not prepared to make any change yet – and 10 represents that you will do everything in your power to try to improve the relationship with your father, what number would you say you're at now? (*Scaling motivation related to the goal*)

FRED: Mmm – oh, I don't know, maybe a 4 or 5.

INTERVIEWER: Good (*Reinforcement, conveys approval*) – so what makes it at least a 4 for you – your willingness to put some effort into this?

FRED: Well, my father is important to me. I do admire him.

Comments: After using a scaling question, a turning point occurs with the discovery of an important client resource – Fred's affection for and even admiration of his father. This resource is unlikely to be apparent either to the interviewer or Fred as long as problem talk persists. When resources or strengths are discovered, it is important to use microquestioning techniques to assertively pursue them and obtain details. When a relationship with another person is a resource to the client, the use of relationship questions is very effective. Observe how the interviewer uses relationship questions related to the dad as well as related to another resource – Fred's mother – to help Fred build a solution.

INTERVIEWER: Oh really! And you even admire him! (*Compliments a potential resource – positive feelings for his father.*)

FRED: Well, yes – he's worked hard all his life and he put my brother and me through school – he sacrificed a lot to give us kids opportunities he didn't have.

INTERVIEWER: Does he know that you admire him – that you appreciate what he's done for you? (*Relationship question*)

FRED: I don't know – I've certainly told my mom.

INTERVIEWER: So, do you think he would appreciate hearing it from you now? (*Displays a curious, not-knowing stance.*)

FRED: Yes, I guess he would, but we don't very often talk like that.

INTERVIEWER: So, it would be unusual for you to talk to your father about feelings? (*Empathy response*)

FRED: Yes, it would be unusual, and it would be hard to do!

INTERVIEWER: Yes, I can see how it might be hard for you (*Empathy response*), but knowing him as well as you do, if you did decide to say something like that (*Pauses here to give Fred time to reflect on this and begin to imagine this happening*), would he see that as a positive gesture on your part – trying to make things better between the two of you? (*Relationship question*)

FRED: I don't know – my father can – yes, probably.

Comment: The interviewer could have asked Fred how his father might see this as helpful; this exploration of the bond between them would likely enhance Fred's determination to follow through. Instead the interviewer pursues another possible resource:

INTERVIEWER: Would your mother say that saying something like that would be helpful to your relationship with your father? (*Relationship question that might create an end-of-session, next-step action plan*)

FRED: Yes, I think she would say it might be helpful, but it'd be really hard for me!

INTERVIEWER: So, she would advise you to try it – she thinks the relationship could stand some improvement? (*Summarizes and repeats the relationship question.*)

FRED: Oh, yes!

INTERVIEWER: Okay, we have only a few minutes left. I think I understand your situation and I would like to give you some feedback about how I see it. Would that be okay?

FRED: Sure.

Feedback and Task Assignment

INTERVIEWER: (*Pauses, takes a deep breath.*) Let me begin by saying how impressed I am with what I see about your family values – how you respect your father and admire him for what he has done for you and your brother. But I understand that there are times when you have been very irritated by your father and you have become so discouraged. I can see how distressing this conflict with your father has been to you, but that you don't want to withdraw from him. (*Pauses and watches to see whether Fred supports this notion.*)

FRED: (*Nods.*)

INTERVIEWER: Your goal of wanting to improve the relationship – I think that's great, but let me check with you again – is that still something you want to do now? (*Checks to see whether the goal is still the same.*)

FRED: Yes, of course.

INTERVIEWER: OK, so I'm wondering whether a good first step for you with your father, if you could do it, and I know you said it would be hard, but if you could actually say something like this to him: that you appreciate all that he has done for you, making the sacrifices he did and so on, and that you would really like to get along better with him. Would that be a good first step?

FRED: Yes I think it might be – if I could talk with my dad that way. And Mother would be pleased – but oh …

INTERVIEWER: Okay, I hear you – but both you and your mother think that this would be good for your relationship with your father and your father would probably respond positively. Right? (*Waits until Fred confirms this.*) On the other hand, you're not sure you are ready yet to have this conversation with your father. Right? (*Fred nods.*) So, here is a tough question for you: when do you think you might be ready to have this conversation with your father?

FRED: (*Long pause*) Well, (*Another long pause*) Thanksgiving is in two weeks. That might be a good time.

INTERVIEWER: Wow – great! (*Complimenting the client*) Knowing your father as well as you do, when do you think might be a good time to approach him on the Thanksgiving weekend?

FRED: Um, ... I don't know. (*Long pause*) Well, after supper, when he goes out for a walk ... Mom doesn't always go with him ... in fact (*Becomes more positive*) I could ask her to let Dad and me go alone ... and I could ask her if Dad had a good day first – she would help me – I can talk to her about most things.

INTERVIEWER: I'm impressed with how well you know your dad – what might work with him – and the good relationship you have with your mom. (*Pause*) So, what would help you make up your mind whether to go through with it – have this talk with your dad?

FRED: (*Pause*) I don't know. (*Another long pause*) You know, I think I'm willing to give it a try after Thanksgiving dinner on Sunday.

INTERVIEWER: That's great – that you care enough about your dad and family, that you're willing to take the first step to try and improve your relationship with your father. I look forward to hearing about how it goes.

FRED: I'll give it a try! I'm feeling good about this!

Note how Fred's affect has changed significantly during the course of the interview. Most solution-focused interviews end in this way, with clients having a much more positive affect and making a strong commitment to follow through on the next-step action plan.

Second and Subsequent Interviews

In follow-up sessions, we begin by asking the client what has become better since our last meeting. If the client (Fred, in this case) brings up the task assignment and it was helpful, we celebrate the success. We might ask, for example, how he was able to do this, what helped him, and what the message of this success is to other challenges in his life. Then we might ask what the client sees as his next step. If he does not raise the subject of the task assignment, we do not usually ask about it. We focus rather on what's working. If the client tells us he tried the task assignment but was unsuccessful, we would inquire about whether the goal is still relevant. If it is, we ask about what needs to happen now for him to reach the goal. If the goal has changed, we go back to goal-phase questions to help the client clarify what is wanted now.

Now let's return to our client Martha from the last chapter and see how the strategy-phase questions are used to promote solution building and how the pastor assigns a next-step action plan. As you may remember, Martha came up with a goal – something she could do that would be helpful to her during this very stressful time.

Example: Martha's Marriage Problem

PASTOR: So, how could you arrange to do that – get away for the weekend, and have time to think? (*Not-knowing question*)

MARTHA: Well – Mom invited me to visit her this weekend, but I didn't want to ask Bill to look after the kids –I didn't want to ask him for anything! But when I think about it –that's silly; it would give me time to think about this mess. And I could visit my best friend Jane – we are very close.

Next-Step Action Plan

PASTOR: Good. Now, is there anything more you want to tell me before I give you some feedback?

MARTHA: No, I think we're OK.

PASTOR: (*Pauses, takes a deep breath.*) Okay, first I want to tell you how impressed I am with how well you're doing at this difficult time. Despite everything, you have made a plan to get away and do some sorting out by going and staying at your mother's. Will it be hard to ask Bill to mind the kids for the weekend? Do we need to talk about that? (*Martha shakes her head.*) So would it be helpful to meet with me early next week, after you've had a chance to get away, and talk to me about this some more?

MARTHA: Oh yes! And you know, I feel so much better now – like things appear more manageable now. I do love Bill, but I've got to think about this more. (*Pause*) Also, I want to thank you for not telling me that I should forgive Bill and get over this. I have to make this decision myself, and I don't really want anyone else's opinion – that's why I didn't call my sister. We are very close, but she would tell me I should "suck it up" because that is what she did.

PASTOR: Okay! Again, in closing, I want to say how much I admire the fact that even through all this pain you feel, you haven't lost sight of what's important to you – your children and family. And I believe you are going to make the best decision when the time is right.

The next and final example illustrates how the solution-focused model addresses a very important problem in health care.

Strategies for Weight Management in a Healthcare Setting

One of our most important public-health concerns today relates to problems resulting from the fact that so many of us are either overweight or obese. The following case example illustrates strength-based, helping strategies that busy healthcare professionals in family medicine can implement within 15 minutes.

Unlike conventional counselling and behaviour-modification approaches to weight loss that emphasize understanding underlying causes, examine past failures, or identify (and seek to modify) current triggers for overeating, the solution-focused model searches for existing strengths and resources that can be utilized to develop patient-specific solutions to weight loss. A major advantage of the solution-focused model is that practitioners can successfully utilize the model's techniques and questions without understanding its development or its theory. Therefore, practitioners can begin right away trying out any of the solution-focused strategies they feel comfortable with. The authors of an excellent article in *Canadian Family Physician* (Greenburg, Ganshorn, & Danilkewich, 2001) state that the biggest obstacle facing family doctors in this regard is that they try initially to do too much, given constraints on time, knowledge, and skill-development, and therefore become discouraged and abandon attempts at using strength-based interventions. These authors encourage physicians to begin using "bits and pieces" of the model and then add to their repertoire of interventions as their experience and comfort grow.

Let's examine how the solution-focused model, using the tri-phase approach, can be used with a patient whose attempts to lose weight over the past few months have not proved successful – despite his having received a referral to a dietician and his having joined Weight Watchers. George comes to his doctor's appointment discouraged. He has reluctantly agreed to a follow-up appointment with his doctor at his wife's urging.

Example: George's Weight Problem

Phase 1 – Establishing Rapport: The doctor acknowledges how hard the client has worked and compliments him on his partial success.

GEORGE: Doctor, I was doing okay for several weeks. Those eating plans from the dietician you recommended helped and I even signed up with Weight Watchers and attended four meetings. I lost ten pounds in that first month and then about three weeks ago I had some problems at work – a fight with my manager. I was so upset that evening when I got home I started snacking again and I lost it! I've been too embarrassed to go back to Weight

Watchers. Now I think I've gained all the weight back. I've just gone back to my old eating habits. I don't dare get on a scale. I don't know what to do. I feel so discouraged!

DOCTOR: I can see how discouraged you are – you were working so hard at it and doing so well and I know you understand how important for your heart condition it is to lose weight. At the same time, I can see how difficult it is for you to lose weight.

GEORGE: Yes, it is! (George goes on to elaborate about how hard he tried and engages in more problem talk. After about a minute, the doctor interrupts.)

DOCTOR: I hear you (*said very sympathetically*), but you were able to lose ten pounds! (*Pauses – patient nods, cautiously agreeing.*) I would really like to know how you were able to do that – to stay on the diet for four weeks.

GEORGE: It was actually closer to five weeks. (*George displays a little more positive affect.*)

DOCTOR: Really! (*Reinforcing*) How did you do that for almost five weeks? It must have been hard.

GEORGE: Yes it was – particularly at first, but you know, once I got started, it seemed to go easier. Those meetings at Weight Watchers helped the most, I think. Hearing how others who were even heavier than me were walking encouraged me to try, by starting small. Also I got a book called *The Step Diet Book*, which included a step counter, so I could see how I increased my steps each day. I really got into it – I was up to 2000 extra steps – a mile – before I crashed. (*George seems more positive.*)

Phase 2 – Goal Settings: George, feeling empowered, recommits himself to his goal of losing weight.

DOCTOR: Yes, that was good, solid progress for you. It sounds like things really worked for you. And you're starting to sound a little more optimistic. I wonder, do you think you might be ready to move forward again on this now?

GEORGE: (*Nods cautiously.*) Yes, I guess so …

DOCTOR: Is that right? Are you really ready to try again?

GEORGE: (*Nods a little more positively.*)

DOCTOR: So, tell me, what is it that tells you that you're ready to try again now?

GEORGE: Well, it's really important to me. I worry about my heart, and for the last while, I have been having more pain. So, I know I have to do it no matter what!

Comments: George responds well to the reinforcement (compliments) on his past success (exceptions strategy) and to the readiness question about starting again, indicating he may be ready to move on to the strategy phase.

Phase 3 – Goal Striving: The doctor helps George work through how he will get back on track.

DOCTOR: So, here is my question for you, George. (*Using the patient's name and saying "my question for you" encourages full attention and effort.*) Knowing yourself as well as you do and all that you have learned about dieting (*Complimenting the patient's past success and efforts*), what do you think is going to work for you? What is one thing that you could do that would begin to get you back on track to losing weight again?

GEORGE: Oh, I don't know. (*A long pause, and the doctor does not interrupt.*) Well, getting back to the step diet – I was on week four of the twelve-week program – that would help. But if I'm going to be honest with myself, I'm probably going to have to go back to Weight Watchers. But I'm not sure I could do that. I'm not sure you can understand, but I'd be so embarrassed. I got to know some of the people there, and everyone was so supportive, and I didn't measure up ...

DOCTOR: I understand it would be embarrassingly hard for you (*Empathy response, pauses*), ... but I want to pick up on this – starting your step diet program again, that would really help, right? (*George nods.*) And if you could do it – get over your embarrassment and return to Weight Watchers – that would help too?

GEORGE: Yes, I think so.

DOCTOR: It sounds like starting the step diet exercise program again and going back to Weight Watchers would help, so what would have to happen for you to be able to get over your embarrassment and go back? (*Outcome question*)

GEORGE: I don't know. (*Long pause and the doctor does not say anything.*) I guess I'd have to swallow my pride – eat humble pie – but that's always been hard for me.

DOCTOR: If you decided you wanted to – how could you swallow your pride in order to start attending Weight Watchers again? What would have to happen? (*Outcome question*)

GEORGE: (*Long pause*) I just have to make up my mind. While we're talking about it, it doesn't seem like such a big deal compared to the risks of not going back.

DOCTOR: *Oh really!* (*Compliment*) Can you say some more about that?

GEORGE: Well – I really want to hang around for a while – I've got things I want to do!

DOCTOR: So reminding yourself you still have things you want to do – that might help you overcome your embarrassment about going back to Weight Watchers? (*Empathy phase*)

GEORGE: (*Nods.*)

DOCTOR: Good. But tell me, what was it about going to Weight Watchers that was so helpful to you? (*Seeking details.*)

GEORGE: I don't know – I think it might be that their point system gave me more choices so I didn't feel so deprived, and the group meetings – that seemed to encourage me – yes, that approach does work for me. And counting my steps every day and only gradually increasing them plus being able to count the steps. I was up to 2000 extra steps a day – that's a mile! I could hardly walk a *block* before I started.

DOCTOR: Great!

Feedback and Task Assignment: The Doctor compliments George and checks to be sure George still wants to go back to Weight Watchers and then assigns a unique task.

DOCTOR: OK. Our time is about up. I want to give you some feedback, OK? (George nods.) First, I want to tell you how pleased I am that your health is so important to you that you want to try the step program again and to overcome your embarrassment about Weight Watchers. And you're considering going back to Weight Watchers – right?"

GEORGE: (*Nods.*)

DOCTOR: And when do you think you might do this?

GEORGE: Well, there is a class tomorrow near where I work, and I like the leader at that one.

DOCTOR: Good! Just one further thing before we finish. I'd like you to think about what you've learned from that conflict with your boss. How do you want to handle it differently when you have another conflict with him in the future? Would you think about that so we can discuss it next month at your visit?

GEORGE: Yes, I will. I don't want to fall off my weight loss plan again!

A Note to the Reader

A cursory reading of this manual might seem to indicate that the solution-focused model consists of a grab bag of techniques and questions. In fact, there are unique and specific techniques and strategies that we use to accomplish our task. Once we begin practising these techniques and strategies, however, we come to realize that the solution-focused model represents a very different way of thinking about clients and how to help them. We look at our clients' capabilities and strengths, and at what's working in their lives, rather than what's wrong. This is a dramatic shift away from exploring the problem. I believe it to be a most respectful way of helping, because, as interviewers, we do not presume to know the answers to our clients' difficulties. Instead, we help our clients to see that by using their strengths and competencies, they can produce their own answers to their difficulties. I also believe that once you begin to practise this model, not only will you think and relate more positively towards others, but you will also increasingly appreciate how your own strengths and successes can support you as you face the inevitable challenges of your own life.

The manual began with a discussion of the power of our questions to create new possibilities, new hope, and new inspiration that can lead to transformation and higher levels of functioning and fulfilment for our clients. The manual will end with a brief discussion of a question that I believe is the most fundamental question of life: "What is the purpose of our brief time on this planet?" Regardless of one's religious or world view, many of us would agree that the answer to this question is somehow related to service to others. What we do with our clients is of the utmost importance. When we help them to see that they have what they need to live their lives with a renewed sense of hope, we are in some way fulfilling our own ultimate purpose. I would like to end with a short quotation that succinctly and poetically captures these thoughts.

Strange is our situation here upon earth.
Each of us comes for a short visit,
not knowing why,
yet sometimes seeming to divine a purpose.
From the standpoint of daily life, however,
there is one thing we do know:
That we are here for the sake of others ...
for the countless unknown souls
with whose fate we are connected
by a bond of sympathy.
Many times a day, I realize
how much my outer and inner life
is built upon the labours of other people,
both living and dead,
and how earnestly I must exert myself
in order to give in return
as much as I have received.

Albert Einstein, from "My Credo" (1932)

Appendix A
SFI Questions: Handy Reference

EMPATHY PHASE: Establishing Rapport

Responses that acknowledge and validate the client, such as
- Simple reinforcements: *Um, Yes, Okay*, etc.
- Repeating the client's words
- Summarizing and reflecting the client's content and affect
- Identifying and complimenting the client's strengths

GOAL-SETTING PHASE: Discovering What's Wanted

- How can I help you?
- What would you like to do (or change) about that?
- How were you hoping I could help you with this problem?

GOAL-STRIVING PHASE: Goal Achieving

1. **Exception Questions: Times When the Problem Doesn't Happen**
   - When doesn't the problem happen?
   - Tell me about the last time you didn't have the problem.
   - What is different about those times?
   - What do you do (or think) differently then?

2. **Outcome Questions: Preferred Future**
   Direct Question
   - When this issue is resolved, or is no longer a problem for you, how will your situation be better for you?

Miracle Question
- Suppose tonight when you go to sleep a miracle happens and this problem is solved. When you wake up tomorrow morning, what would be different? How would you be different? What would others notice?

3. Scaling Questions: Assessment Technique
- Using a scale of 1 to 10, where 1 is the worst (lowest) things have been for you, and 10 is where the problem is resolved (you reach your goal), where would you rate your confidence (problem, self-esteem) right now?
- How important is it to you to make these changes? Using a scale of 1 to 10, where 1 is that you aren't ready to do anything yet, and 10 is that you will do everything possible, what number would you choose?

4. Relationship Questions: Soliciting Other Opinions
- What would your wife (husband) say has to happen for her (him) to take you back in the marriage?
- What would your wife (father, friend, doctor) say is the reason she (he) sent you to see me?
- What would (that person) need to see for her (him) to believe you don't need to come here anymore?

5. Coping Questions: Survival Tactics
- How have you managed to cope as well as you have with that problem?
- What have you done to keep this situation from becoming worse?

Appendix B
Brief Post-Traumatic Growth Rating Scale

Using a scale of 0 to 5, rate the following items in terms of being affected by an extreme life adversity (trauma):

(a) I have a greater appreciation of my own life   ____
(b) I have discovered that I am stronger than I thought   ____
(c) I have established a new path for my life   ____
(d) I have a greater sense of closeness with others   ____
(e) I have a greater understanding of spiritual matters   ____

Total Score = ____

(Adapted from Seligman, M. (2011), a comprehensive summary of the science of positive psychology.)

I use the simplified version above by asking clients or group members to complete the rating scale and talk about the items with the highest scores, providing specific details about all the ways they have benefited from their adverse experience(s). For more information about PTG see chapter 4.

Background: US Army's Comprehensive Soldier Fitness Program and Post-Traumatic Growth

To put it quite simply, post-traumatic growth (PTG) is a higher level of psychological functioning achieved as a result of surviving a trauma or other extreme adversity. The evidence supporting PTG and resiliency training was sufficiently convincing that the US Army has created the Comprehensive Soldier Fitness program (CSF; see http://csf.army

.mil). A central part of the CSF is the well-established Post-Traumatic Growth Inventory, which assesses growth in (a) to (e) above. (To see the full version, visit http://cust-cf.apa.org/ptgi.)

Appendix C
Training and Certification Opportunities

As a result of the tireless efforts of Insoo Kim Berg, Steve de Shazer, and their colleagues, there are today many excellent opportunities around the world to learn the solution-focused approach. The University of Toronto, in 1999, was one of the first universities to offer a comprehensive, specialist-level, solution-focused training program at the graduate level.

University of Toronto Solution-Focused Programs

The certificate program in Solution-Focused Counselling begun in 1999, is offered through the Faculty of Social Work and is intended to teach solution-building skills at the specialist level. The program consists of six two-day modules for a total of 72 classroom hours, and is directed at professionals in such human service fields as counselling, social work, psychology, nursing, and medicine.

In 2010 a Solution-Focused Coaching stream was launched responding to the rapidly growing field of professional coaching – from life coaching to executive coaching – using a similar modular format and an experiential learning structure such as live coaching. The coaching program features international leaders in solution-focused community and interdisciplinary communities such as Peter Szabo (Switzerland), Fredrike Bannink (Netherlands), and Simon Lee (Singapore). The program is directed at professionals in HR, knowledge management, leadership, and organizational development, both in the public and private sectors. Students may take up to two modules from either stream.

More information about the solution-focused programs is available from the University of Toronto, Faculty of Social Work, Continuing Education Coordinator. Email: fsw.conted@utoronto.ca. Voicemail: 416-978-3259. Website: http://www.socialwork.utoronto.ca/conted/certificate/solfocus.htm.

Canadian Council of Professional Certification

In 1975, the Canadian Council of Professional Certification (CCPC) was granted a federal charter for the purpose of recognizing the accomplishments of professionals working in their specific disciplines. Since its inception, the CCPC has granted certification to professionals in a wide variety of disciplines: addiction counsellors, gambling counsellors, community service workers, solution-focused specialists, and business managers, among others. The CCPC is unique in that its federal charter is not restricted to recognizing Canadian residents. The wording of the charter explicitly permits it to extend its recognition beyond Canada. A new logo, CCPC GLOBAL, was adopted in 2009 to reflect the participation of the CCPC in the global market

Background of the Development of the Solution-Focused Credentials

Some of the early graduates of the U of T program expressed interest in pursuing professional recognition beyond the university level. On behalf of these students, Dr Warner made an application to the board of directors of the CCPC to establish a solution-focused specialist-level certification. In 2001, that board created a new professional designation – Certified Solution-Focused Therapist (CSFT) – using for its standards the U of T Solution-Focused Counselling Certificate Program. In addition to requiring the completion of 72 hours of classroom or workshop training, the CCPC mandated the completion of a supervision component for this certification.

Although the U of T Solution-Focused Counselling Program was originally intended for counsellors and therapists, other helping professionals, including healthcare providers, educators, human resource specialists, and life coaches, began attending classes. These helping professionals also expressed interest in obtaining CCPC certification. The CCPC therefore created two other solution-focused professional designations – the CSFP (Practitioner) and CSFC (Coach). Interest in these solution-focused certifications has been steadily growing both within Canada and abroad. In addition to Canadians, the CCPC has awarded solution-focused certification to professionals in England, Scotland, Poland, Malaysia, the Philippines, and Singapore.

In addition to the above-mentioned U of T training program, there are currently approved training centres in Eastern and Western Canada, and three international academies. For more information and an up-to-date listing, visit the CCPC website.

The addresses for the Canadian Council of Professional Certification are as follows:

Head Office:
1 Edenmills Drive, Toronto, Ontario, Canada M1E 4L1
Tel.: 416-724-5339; Fax: 416-724-0884
E-mail: info@ccpcglobal.com
Website: www.ccpcglobal.com

Western Canada Office:
3404–3000 Somervale Court SW, Calgary, Alberta, Canada T2Y 4J2
Tel.: 403-201-2123
E-mail: wco@ccpcglobal.com

Appendix D
A Paradigm Shift: My Journey

Little did I realize almost three decades ago that my pursuit of skills in a particular brief therapy model would lead me to abandon one of psychology's central assumptions – I would discard the belief that assessment and diagnosis of client problems and subsequent expert-driven solutions and treatment planning are of critical importance to psychotherapeutic effectiveness. (This is not a new position – Carl Rogers had been writing about that since the 1950s; see Rogers, 1959.) And more recent research, in a five-year follow-up study by Gibbard and Hanley (2008), indicates that "person-centred counselling is effective for clients with common mental health problems, such as anxiety and depression. Effectiveness is not limited to individuals with mild to moderate symptoms of recent onset, but extends to people with moderate to severe symptoms of longer duration" (p. 215).

An Eclectic Beginning

For the first 20 years I spent as a counselling psychologist at Ryerson University's Centre for Student Development and Counselling, my theoretical orientation was eclectic. This approach appealed to me because I could choose from the best practices of all theoretical orientations. Using Gestalt techniques, for example, I would encourage clients to "get into their feelings," and although the process was sometimes slow, I was generally quite satisfied with the results. However, with increasing demands for accountability and the new emphasis on "downsizing" that began to emerge in the late 1980s, it became apparent to me that I was going to have to make changes to my professional practice. The luxury of offering time-unlimited, humanistic-oriented counselling to my university-student clients was becoming out of step with the new reality. Although the mean number of my university counselling sessions was six, I had treated some of my student clients for a year or longer. As I look back, I realize that many of these long-term counselling relationships took on a mentoring quality. Although I believe these relationships still had therapeutic value for my clients, and were certainly satisfying to me, the resource utilization left room for improvement.

What also fostered my thinking about the potential to accomplish more in less time was a book by Moshe Talmon (1990) that I discovered at an Ontario Psychology Association convention book display. I was attracted to the book because of its seemingly ridiculous title – *Single-Session Therapy: Maximizing the Effect of the First (and Often Only) Therapeutic Encounter*. Talmon made two compelling points in this book that were going to influence my research agenda. The first was that there is considerable evidence that the single psychotherapeutic session is the most common (modal) length of treatment. The second was that follow-up studies consistently find that the majority of those clients who only attend one session are satisfied and do not return because they got what they wanted.

After reading Talmon's book, I began to explore brief therapy models, including solution-focused brief therapy. This did not mean that I was ready to give up my favourite intervention – "How does that make you feel?" – and my other emotionally intensifying techniques. What it did mean, however, was that I was becoming more convinced of how important a role cognition and behaviour play in the therapeutic process.

Becoming Solution-Focused in My Practice

My first learning experience with SFBT occurred in 1990, when I attended a one-day workshop taught by SFBT co-founder Steve de Shazer. Although I was not overly impressed by the taped interviews that were shown (little attention was paid to client affect), I found many of the ideas and techniques interesting and practical. Towards the end of the workshop I asked the question, "How can the solution to a problem be independent of that problem?" This concept seemed so counter-intuitive to all my training and experience. I remember de Shazer looking at me, scratching his head and saying, "That's what this whole workshop has been about!" Well, I didn't "get it."

For quite some time after the workshop (at least two years) I continued to grapple with the question of how the solutions to clients' difficulties could be independent of their presenting problems. In spite of my scepticism, I started using some of the techniques of SFBT, very timidly at first. But as my clients started talking about the progress they were making between sessions, I became increasingly convinced of the potential of this model. I started extending the interval between client visits from one week to two weeks (with the clear understanding that I was available earlier if necessary). As I continued to take training in SFBT, my skill in applying the model grew. By the early 1990s I would have described myself as eclectic with a preference for SFBT – I used it about half the time. When I got stuck, I reverted to the problem-centred approach. This is typical of intermediate skill development in the practice of SFBT.

One of the things that helped build my confidence that the SFBT approach in and of itself was sufficient for my practice and that I did not need to fall back on problem-based interventions was learning to teach the SFBT model. At this time I was an adjunct professor in the Counselling Psychology Program at OISE/Toronto, teaching a variety of psychology courses that helped me keep up to date on theoretical orientations. Because of my interest in brief therapies, I proposed (to the chair of the Psychology Department, Dr Mary Alice Guttman) offering a "Brief Counselling Strategies" course that would survey the various brief therapy models, including both cognitive-behavioural and emotionally based approaches. The chair indicated that she preferred a more practice-oriented course for students. I was not particularly happy with her decision, as this would involve more work than I had planned on doing. The larger practice component of the course required, I felt, a more in-depth background, and so I sought out more training and supervision to enhance my brief therapy skills. I was becoming more immersed in the SFBT model.

An example of how far I had changed in my practice was that I now rarely asked clients, "How do you feel?" but rather asked, "How are you doing?" This is a subtle but important shift and was reflective of my movement away from emotionally based interventions. Trusting that my clients really did have the answers to their problems permitted me to adopt a "not-knowing, non-expert" posture, and this in turn helped my clients to create their own solutions more quickly. The mean number of my client sessions was eventually reduced by half (from six to three). Although my client load increased, I was no longer as tired by Friday afternoon as I had been when I saw fewer clients but used a problem-centred approach. I became interested in the question of whether, with briefer treatments, students were being well served. This led me to undertake a year-long outcome study of clients who sought personal counselling at Ryerson University. The results of this study (involving three counsellors) indicated that clients were equally satisfied with the service received regardless of the number of sessions they attended (Warner, 1996a – see chapter 2 above for more details).

Providing Continuing Education for Helping Professionals

During the last five years before I took early retirement from Ryerson, I was provided with the wonderful opportunity (thanks to Marion Creery, the director of student services) of offering my services as a solution-focused trainer to mental-health professionals in hospitals and community clinics. I also began making annual visits to the Centre for Studies in Counselling at the University of Durham (UK), where I offered workshops and made presentations on brief therapy topics, and where I was made an honorary research fellow. Teaching these SFBT workshops has been very gratifying to me. The feedback I frequently receive from workshop participants is that this training challenges them to see their clients from a competency perspective and affects not only their professional practice but their personal lives as well. For example, psychiatric nurses, social workers, and other healthcare practitioners at two Toronto-area hospitals reported increased levels of job satisfaction and skill development as well as enhanced ability to handle a wide range of patient problems as a result of solution-focused training (Warner, 1998). Similar professional development benefits were found with childcare workers (Triantafillou, 1997; Warner, 1997), rehabilitation professionals (Warner, 2001), and public health nurses (Bowman, 2003).

My two-day SFBT workshops were titled "Basic Skills" and I offered them to a wide range of helping professionals. The relevance of this strength-based training is reflected in the fact that the following credentialling organizations approved 12 hours of continuing education credits for the workshops: the College of Family Physicians of Canada, the Ontario College of Social Workers, the Commission of Rehabilitation Counselling, the Ontario College of Teachers, and the Canadian Council of Professional Certification. This early version of my Basic Skills workshop has now been incorporated into the Solution-Focused Counselling certificate program at the Faculty of Social Work of the University of Toronto.

University of Toronto Solution-Focused Training Program

In 1998 I had the honour of being invited to set up a certificate program in SFBT at the University of Toronto in the Faculty of Social Work. The U of T was one of the first universities to offer a comprehensive solution-focused specialist-level training program. When the program began, I was uncertain whether there was sufficient interest in the professional community to sustain a one-year, solution-focused specialist-level program. I am pleased to report that after almost a decade and a half, the counselling program continues to flourish. In 2012 the number of graduates of the program was close to 300, and it is because of their success and their recommendations to others that the program is thriving. Four of the graduates are now part of the teaching faculty, educating the next generation of practitioners. In 2010 we added a solution-focused coaching program, and even in this short time, the coaching program has been able to attract instructors who are some of the leading international trainers in the solution-focused community (see appendix C for more details).

When I reflect on two decades of teaching students in the Counselling Psychology Program and at the Faculty of Social Work at the U of T, I recall with pride the many I have mentored who have used their solution-focused, strength-based skills to make a difference in their communities. Two of my former students, Jason Kelly and Haesun Moon, however, I would like to acknowledge. They were so committed to deepening their understanding of this approach that they wanted to learn directly from the leaders in the solution-focused field. This was reflected in their attending solution-focused conferences and training sessions that required travelling to the United States, Europe, and the Far East. The older one, a remarkable young man, Jason Kelly, was setting up his addictions counselling practice in Thailand, and was consulting with me about setting up an Internet therapy service. On a return trip to Thailand, after we had discussed collaborating on a book together, Jason died of a stroke at thirty-seven years of age. Thanks to the generosity of his family, however, the Jason Kelly Leadership Award was established, and once a year we celebrate his memory and acknowledge a graduate who has made a significant contribution to his or her community. To date we have the bestowed the Jason Kelly Leadership Award upon five recipients.

The first recipient of the Jason Kelly Leadership Award was Haesun Moon. When Jason visited me on one of his trips from the Far East, I introduced him to Haesun at a lunch meeting, and it turned out that he was able to facilitate a unique coaching supervision placement for her. Haesun went on to rapidly advance her career, collaborating with some of the leading solution-focused practitioners. When the Solution-Focused Coaching program was launched in 2010, she was my first recommendation for the position of program director. With the visiting lecturers she has been able to attract, the program is gaining an international reputation and has become considerably enriched and inspiring to the next generation of solution-focused coaches. She has exceeded my expectations.

Having the privilege of influencing the next generation of professionals has been one of the most rewarding and satisfying experiences of my career.

References

American Psychological Association. (2009). *The post-traumatic inventory: The road to resilience*. Retrieved November 2012 from www.apa.org.

Australian Psychological Society. (2003). *Coaching psychology interest group mission statement*. Retrieved November 2003 from www.groups.psychology.org.au/igcp.

Bannick, F.P. (2014). *Posttraumatic success: Solution-focused and positive psychology strategies to help clients survive and thrive after trauma*. New York: Norton.

Bavelas, J.B., McGee, D., Phillips, B., & Routledge, R. (2000). Microanalysis of communication in psychotherapy. *Human Systems: The Journal of Systemic Consultation and Management, 11*(1), 47–66.

Berg, I. (1992). Irreconcilable differences: A solution-focused approach to marital therapy. Videotape. Available from www.brief-therapy.org.

Berg, I. (1994). *Family based services: A solution-focused approach*. New York: Norton.

Berg, I., & Miller, S. (1992). *Working with the problem drinker: A solution-focused approach*. New York, London: Norton.

Berg, I., & Reuss, N. (1997). *Solutions step by step: A substance abuse treatment manual*. New York: Norton.

Berg, I., & Szabo, P. (2005). *Brief coaching for lasting solutions*. New York: Norton.

Bergin, A., & Garfield, S. (1994). *Manual of psychotherapy and behaviour change* (4th ed.). New York: Wiley & Sons.

Bloom, B. L. (1992). *Planned short-term psychotherapy: A clinical manual*. New York: Allyn & Bacon.

Bohart, A., & Tallman, K. (1999). *How clients make therapy work: The process of active self-healing*. Washington: American Psychological Association.

Bowman, V. (2003). "An evaluation of the training of public health nurses and family visitors in the use of brief solution-focused interview methods." Unpublished report, York Region Health Services.

Branan, J. (1972). Negative human interaction. *Journal of Counselling Psychology, 19*(1), 82–83.

Cook, J. (2007). The top ten most influential therapists of the past quarter-century. *Psychotherapy Networker* (March/April), 24–37.

Costello, S. (2003). "A microanalysis of Insoo Kim Berg's interventions [in] irreconcilable differences: A solution-focused approach to marital therapy" [Videotape]. Unpublished paper, University of Toronto, available from the author.

De Jong, P., & Berg, I. (2008). *Interviewing for solutions*. New York: Brooks/Cole.

de Shazer, S. (1985). *Keys to solution in brief therapy*. New York: Norton.

de Shazer, S. (1988). *Clues: Investigating solutions in brief therapy*. New York: Norton.

de Shazer, S. (1991). *Putting difference to work*. New York: Norton.

Duncan, B., & Miller, S. (2000). *The heroic client*. San Francisco: Jossey- Bass.

Duncan, B., Miller, S., Wampold, B., & Hubble, M. (Eds.). (2009). *The heart & soul of change: Delivering what works in therapy*. American Psychological Association. Washington, DC.

Easton, M. (2005). What makes us happy: Science offers surprising answers. *University of Toronto Magazine, 32*(1) (Spring), 20–26.

Fiske, H. (2008). *Hope in action: Solution-focused conversations about suicide*. London: Routledge.

Franklin, C., Trepper, T., Gingerich, W., & McCollum, E. (Eds.). (2012). *Solution-focused brief therapy: A manual of evidence-based practice*. Oxford University Press.

Fredrickson, B., & Losada, M. (2005). Positive affect and the complex dynamics of human flourishing. *American Psychologist, 60*(7), 678–686.

Gable, S.L., Reis, H.T., Impett, E.A., & Asher, R.R. (2004). What do you do when things go right? The intrapersonal and interpersonal benefits of sharing good events. *Journal of Personality and Social Psychology, 87*, 228–245.

Gibbard, I., & Hanley, T. (2008). A five-year evaluation of the effectiveness of person-centred counselling in routine clinical practice in primary care. *Counselling and Psychotherapy Research, 8*(4) (December), 215–222.

Gingerich, W. J., & Eisengart, S. (2000). Solution-focused brief therapy: A review of the outcome research. *Family Process, 39*, 477–498.

Glassman, D., & Grawe, K. (2006). General change mechanisms: The relation between problem activation and resource activation in successful and unsuccessful therapeutic interactions. *Clinical Psychology and Psychotherapy, 13*, 1–11.

Gottman, J.M., & Krokoff, L.J. (1989). The relationship between marital interaction and marital satisfaction: A longitudinal view. *Journal of Consulting
and Clinical Psychology, 57,* 47–52.

Grant, A., & Greene, J. (2001). *Coach yourself: Make real change in your life.* Cam-
bridge, MA: Perseus Publishing.

Green, L.S., Oades, L.G., & Grant, A.M. (2006). Cognitive-behavioural, solution-focused life coaching: Enhancing goal striving, well-being, and hope.
Journal of Positive Psychology, 1(3), 142–149.

Green, S. (2012). Solution-focused life coaching. In Franklin, Trepper, Gingerich, & McCollum (Eds.), *Solution-focused brief therapy: A manual of evidence-based practice.* Oxford University Press.

Greenberg, G., Ganshorn, K., & Danilkewich, A. (2001). Solution-focused
therapy: Counselling model for busy family physicians. *Canadian Family
Physician, 47,* 2289–2295.

Greene, G., & Lee, M. (2011). *Solution-oriented social work practice.* Oxford University Press.

Hubble, M.A., Duncan, B.L., & Miller, S.D. (1999). *The heart and soul of change.*
Washington: APA Press.

Johnson, L., & Miller, S. (1994). Modification of depression risk factors: A solution-focused approach. *Psychotherapy, 31*(3), 244–253.

Joseph, S., & Linley, A. (2006). *Positive therapy: A meta-theory for positive psychological practice.* London: Routledge.

Joseph, S., & Linley, A. (2008). *Trauma, recovery, and growth: Positive psychological perspectives on post-traumatic stress.* John Wiley & Sons.

Losada, M. (1999). "The complex dynamics of high performance teams."
Mathematical and Computer Modelling, 30(9–10), 179–192.

McGee, D. (1999). Constructive questions: How do therapeutic questions
work? Unpublished doctoral dissertation, Department of Psychology, University of Victoria, BC, Canada.

McGee, D., Del Vento, A., & Bavelas, J. (2005). An interactional model of questions as therapeutic interventions. *Journal of Marital and Family Therapy,
31*(4), 371–384.

McKay, K., Imel, Z., & Wampold, B. (2006). Psychiatrist effects in the psychopharmacological treatment of depression. *Journal of Affective Disorders, 92*(2),
287–290.

Rachlis, M. (2004). *Prescriptions for excellence: How innovation is saving Canada's
healthcare system.* New York: HarperCollins.

Rath, T., & Clifton, D. (2004). *How full is your bucket? Positive strategies for work
and life.* New York: Gallup Press.

Rogers, C.R. (1959). A theory of therapy, personality, and interpersonal relations, as developed in the client-centred framework. In S. Koch (Ed.), *Psychology: A study of science*, vol. 3. New York: McGraw-Hill.

Seligman, M. (1998). Building human strength: Psychology's forgotten missions. *American Psychological Association Monitor*, January, 2–20.

Seligman, M. (2002). *Authentic happiness: Using the new positive psychology*. New York: Free Press.

Seligman, M. (2011). *Flourish: A new understanding of happiness and well-being*. New York: Free Press.

Seligman, M., & Fowler, R. (2011). Comprehensive soldier fitness and the future of psychology. *American Psychologist, 66*(1), 82–86.

Sklare, G. (2005). *Brief counselling that works: A solution-focused approach for school counsellors and administrators*. Thousand Oaks, CA: Corwin Press.

Smith, D. (1982). Trends in counselling and psychotherapy. *American Psychologist, 37*, 802–809.

Steenbarger, B.N. (1994). Duration and outcome in psychotherapy: An integrative review. *Professional Psychology: Research and Practice, 25*, 111–119.

Talley, J. (1992). *The predictors of successful very brief psychotherapy: A study of differences by gender, age, and treatment variables*. New York: C. C. Thomas.

Talmon, M. (1990). *Single-session therapy: Maximizing the effect of the first (and often only) therapeutic encounter*. San Francisco: Jossey-Bass.

Tedeschi, R. (2011). Posttraumatic growth in combat veterans. *J Clin Psychol Med Settings, 18*, 137–144.

Tedeschi, R., & Calhoun, L. (1996). The posttraumatic growth inventory: Measuring the positive legacy of trauma. *Journal of Traumatic Stress, 9*, 455–471.

Tomori, C., & Bavelas, J. (2007). Using microanalysis of communication to compare solution-focused and client-centred therapies. *Journal of Family Psychotherapies, 18*(3), 25–43.

Triantafillou, N. (1997). A solution-focused approach to mental health supervision. *Journal of Systemic Therapy, 16*(4), 305–328.

US Army. (2012). Longitudinal analysis of the impact of master resilience training on self-reported resilience and psychological health data. Report #3 (internal document). Most recent CSF evaluation.

Wade, A. (1997). Small acts of living: Everyday resistance to violence and other forms of oppression. *Contemporary Family Therapy, 19*, 23–40.

Wade, A. (2000). Resistance to personal violence: Implications for the practice of therapy. Unpublished doctoral dissertation, Department of Psychology, University of Victoria, Victoria, BC, Canada.

Wallis, C. (2005, January 9). The new science of happiness. *Time Magazine*, 39–85.

Walter, J., & Peller, J. (1992). *Becoming solution-focused in brief therapy*. New York: Brunner/Mazel.

Wampold, B. (2001). *The great psychotherapy debate: Models, methods, and findings*. Lawrence Erlbaum.

Warner, R.E. (1989). The most negative life experiences of the elderly. *Canadian Social Work Review, 6*(2), 176–185.

Warner, R.E. (1990). The most negative life experiences of college students. *Canadian Journal of Counselling, 23*(1), 36–44.

Warner, R.E. (1991a). Canadian university counsellors: A survey of theoretical orientations and other related descriptors. *Canadian Journal of Counselling, 25*(1), 33–37.

Warner, R.E. (1991b). A survey of theoretical orientations of Canadian clinical psychologists. *Canadian Psychology, 32*(3), 525–528.

Warner, R.E. (1996a). Comparison of client and counsellor satisfaction with treatment duration. *Journal of College Student Psychotherapy, 10*(3), 73–88.

Warner, R.E. (1996b). Counsellor bias against shorter-term counselling: A comparison of counsellor and client satisfaction in a Canadian setting. *International Journal for the Advancement of Counselling, 18*, 1–10.

Warner, R.E. (1997). Implementing the solution-focused model: One therapist's experience. *Journal of Collaborative Therapies, 5*(1), 8–14.

Warner, R.E. (1998). Mental health services staff training in hospital settings: A solution-focused approach. *Partners in Psychiatric Health Care, 1*(1), 32–37.

Warner, R.E. (2001). The solution-focused approach to rehabilitation counselling. *Canadian Rehab Review*, (Fall), 35–36.

Warner, R.E. (2012). Strength thorough adversity: Promoting post-traumatic growth strategies. A presentation to the Canadian Institute of Military and Veterans Health Research Forum, Queen's University.